Sun, skin and health

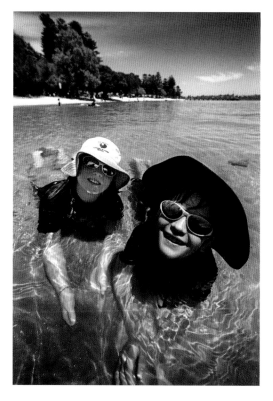

Edited by Terry Slevin

CSIRO

PUBLISHING

National Library of Australia Cataloguing-in-Publication entry

Sun, skin and health/editor: Terry Slevin.

9781486301157 (paperback)
9781486301164 (ebook)
9781486301171 (ebook)

Includes bibliographical references and index.

Skin – Cancer – Australia – Prevention.
Skin – Cancer – Treatment – Australia.
Skin – Protection – Australia.

Slevin, Terry, editor.

616.99477

Published by
CSIRO Publishing
150 Oxford Street (PO Box 1139)
Collingwood VIC 3066
Australia

Telephone: +61 3 9662 7666
Local call: 1300 788 000 (Australia only)
Fax: +61 3 9662 7555
Email: publishing.sales@csiro.au
Website: www.publish.csiro.au

Front cover (background): fotopike/Shutterstock.com
Front cover (left to right): courtesy Queensland Health; with permission of Cancer Council Western Australia; courtesy Community Newspaper Group
Title page: © *The West Australian*
Back cover (left to right): © *The West Australian*; aslysun/Shutterstock.com

Figures are by the relevant chapter author unless noted otherwise.

Set in 10.5/16 Adobe Minion Pro and Optima
Edited by Adrienne de Kretser, Righting Writing
Cover design by Andrew Weatherill
Typeset by Desktop Concepts Pty Ltd, Melbourne
Index by Master Indexing
Printed in China by 1010 Printing International Ltd

CSIRO Publishing publishes and distributes scientific, technical and health science books, magazines and journals from Australia to a worldwide audience and conducts these activities autonomously from the research activities of the Commonwealth Scientific and Industrial Research Organisation (CSIRO). The views expressed in this publication are those of the author(s) and do not necessarily represent those of, and should not be attributed to, the publisher or CSIRO. The copyright owner shall not be liable for technical or other errors or omissions contained herein. The reader/user accepts all risks and responsibility for losses, damages, costs and other consequences resulting directly or indirectly from using this information.

Original print edition:
The paper this book is printed on is in accordance with the rules of the Forest Stewardship Council®. The FSC® promotes environmentally responsible, socially beneficial and economically viable management of the world's forests.

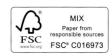

Royalties from the sale of this book will be donated to the Cancer Council Western Australia.

Foreword

It's tough being a fair-skinned person in Australia. We love sunshine and there are many beautiful places to enjoy it. Our incomes, that are high by global standards, make it easier for us to get out on the waters of our oceans and to enjoy holidays in sunny places. But all this potential for fun in the sun is spoiled by ever-present warnings about cancers that enjoying the sun might cause.

Each year Australians are treated for upward of 750 000 cancers caused by sun exposure, almost all skin cancers. Not so daunting, but more frightening, are the 2000 or so Australians who die each year from sun-caused cancers; the TV reminds us that some killed are in their 20s and 30s.

These dark sides of the sun are real. We can't ignore them but we can adapt to them; knowledge is the key to adaptation.

I'm lucky. I've been a participant in growing knowledge about the sun and health for 40 years. Knowing how to enjoy the sun and protect myself against skin cancer is 'in my bones'. But it really isn't all that difficult.

First, when making decisions about sun protection, I take account of where I am, the season and the time of day. I am much more careful when I am in a low-latitude place (most of Australia), it's summer and I intend going out in the middle of the day. Together, these three tell me that there will be high levels of cancer-causing ultraviolet (UV) rays in sunshine. Putting the three factors together for anywhere, any season and any time can be challenging, and that's where the daily UV Index forecast comes in handy; you'll find it with the weather forecast in most Australian newspapers. When the UV Index is going to be less than 3, I don't bother with sun protection. When it's going to be higher and I'll be outside for more than a few minutes here and there, I do.

Second, clothing is the best protection: I cover as much of my skin as practical given the forecast temperature and what I intend doing. I protect the skin of my face with a broad-brimmed hat. Protecting your face is very important; skin cancers are common there and it's the place you'd least like to have one treated.

Third, I apply an SPF30+ broad-spectrum sunscreen to any skin that's still exposed, including my face; I don't just depend on the hat. If you plan ahead, it's much easier to do this immediately after drying yourself from the morning shower. You don't get the sunscreen on your clothes and you're less likely to miss bits of skin that will be exposed. Don't forget the top of your feet if you're wearing sandals, and the backs of your hands – these are very susceptible to some skin cancers.

Fourth, get into shade whenever it's available and fits with what you want to do. It's a great way to reduce the UV Index where you are.

I can hear you ask, 'What about vitamin D?' I aim to have some outdoor time and not use sun protection when the UV Index is under 3. Walking for part of both ends of the daily commute, or other early morning or late afternoon activities, is an easy way to get some vitamin D.

Simple, but there is 40 years of experience behind this advice. By reading this book you can gain the benefit of hundreds of years of experience of experts on sun and health. The best cook is not one who can just read and follow a recipe, like my sun protection recipe, but one who understands what works in preparing great food and how best to do it. Food, sun – we should enjoy them both.

Bruce Armstrong AM FAA
Emeritus Professor
Sydney School of Public Health
The University of Sydney

Contents

Acknowledgements

Books never happen without enormous effort and patience from lots of people.

My chapter authors have been a joy to work with, generous of their time and expertise. All are stand out experts in their field who work very hard to establish and maintain their expertise. All did much or all of this extra work in their 'spare time'. To them all I am extremely grateful. I offer one special note of thanks to Peter Gies – as he led the charge on not one but two important chapters in the book.

The Cancer Council 'Family' have been vital in getting this book over the line. Special thanks to all my mates at Cancer Councils, particularly those at Cancer Council Victoria and Cancer Council Australia. All these people are dedicated to making an impact on this mongrel of a disease and their dedication is admirable, remarkable and exemplary.

My own crew at Cancer Council Western Australia have not only been very helpful, they have also put up with me as looming deadlines have meant other things have been ignored and the temperature has risen. Karola Belohradsky, Lindsey Orton and Anna Nankivell have all made vital contributions. So too have the 'SunSmarties' in the form of Mark Strickland and Carolyn Minto.

The crew at CSIRO Publishing have guided me as a 'first timer' and have been great. Special thanks to Julia Stuthe, Tracey Millen and Lauren Webb.

I want to pay special tribute to Clive Deverall. Clive was the pioneer of Cancer Council's affordable range of sun protection merchandise. It is hard to imagine the modern skin cancer prevention efforts without Clive's early leadership in the field. Thanks also to the MPDS.

Most of all I dedicate this book to my family who continue to let me get away with too much. Jenelle, Nicki, Pat and of course my mum – thanks and I love you.

List of contributors

Jonathan Chan MBBS FACD. Consultant Dermatologist, Sir Charles Gairdner Hospital, Nedlands WA 6009.

Alvin Chong MBBS, MMed, FACD. Senior Lecturer and Consultant Dermatologist, Skin and Cancer Foundation Inc., St Vincent's Hospital Melbourne, University of Melbourne, 80 Drummond St, Carlton Vic. 3053.

Judith Cole MB BS MPH FACD. Consultant Dermatologist, St John of God Dermatology, Subiaco WA 6008.

Minas Coroneo BSc (Med) MBBS MSc MD MS FRACS FRANZCO. Professor and Chairman, Department of Ophthalmology, University of New South Wales, Sydney NSW 2052.

Stephen Dain BSc PhD FCOptom FAAO FIES (ANZ) FMSA. Director, Optics and Radiometry Laboratory, and Professor, School of Optometry and Vision Science, University of New South Wales, Sydney NSW 2052.

Brian Diffey BSc AKC PhD DSc. Emeritus Professor of Photobiology, Dermatological Sciences, Institute of Cellular Medicine, Newcastle University NE2 4HH, UK.

Suzanne Dobbinson PhD. Senior Research Fellow, Cancer Council Victoria, 615 St Kilda Rd, Melbourne Vic. 3004.

Kimberley Dunstone BSc (Hons). SunSmart Research and Evaluation Officer, Centre for Behavioural Research in Cancer, Cancer Council Victoria, 615 St Kilda Rd, Melbourne Vic. 3004.

Jon Emery MA MBBCh FRACGP MRCGP DPhil. Herman Professor of Primary Care Cancer Research, University of Melbourne. General Practice and Primary Care Academic Centre, 200 Berkeley St, Carlton Vic. 3053.

Peter Foley MBBS BMedSci MD FACD. Associate Professor and Director of Research, Skin and Cancer Foundation Inc., University of Melbourne, 80 Drummond St, Carlton Vic. 3053.

Peter Gies PhD. Senior Research Scientist, UVR Group, Non Ionising Radiation Section, Radiation Health Services Branch, Australian Radiation Protection and Nuclear Safety Agency, 619 Lower Plenty Rd, Yallambie Vic. 3085.

Stuart Henderson PhD. Scientist, UVR Group, Non Ionising Radiation Section, Radiation Health Services Branch, Australian Radiation Protection and Nuclear Safety Agency, 619 Lower Plenty Rd, Yallambie Vic. 3085.

John Javorniczky PhD. Scientist, UVR Group, Non Ionizing Radiation Section, Radiation Health Services Branch, Australian Radiation Protection and Nuclear Safety Agency, 619 Lower Plenty Rd, Yallambie Vic. 3085.

Kerryn King PhD. Scientist, UVR Group, Non Ionising Radiation Section, Radiation Health Services Branch, Australian Radiation Protection and Nuclear Safety Agency, 619 Lower Plenty Rd, Yallambie Vic. 3085.

Robyn M Lucas MBChB PhD. Winthrop Professor and Research Strategy Leader, Telethon Kids Institute, 100 Roberts Rd, Subiaco WA 6008. Professor and Head, Environment, Climate and Health, National Centre for Epidemiology and Population Health, The Australian National University, Canberra ACT 0200.

Christina Mackay BArch MBA FNZIA. Registered Architect. Senior Lecturer, School of Architecture, Faculty of Architecture and Design, Victoria University of Wellington, PO Box 600, Wellington NZ.

Jen Makin MSc. Program Manager Sense-T, University of Tasmania, Churchill Ave, Sandy Bay Tas. 7005.

Alan McLennan UVR Group, Non Ionizing Radiation Section, Radiation Health Services Branch, Australian Radiation Protection and Nuclear Safety Agency, 619 Lower Plenty Rd, Yallambie Vic. 3085.

Rachel Neale BVSC PhD. Head, Cancer Aetiology and Prevention Group, QIMR Berghofer Medical Research Institute, 300 Herston Rd, Herston Qld 4006.

Catherine Olsen BSc (Hons I) PhD MPH. Senior Research Officer, Cancer Control Group, QIMR Berghofer Medical Research Institute, 300 Herston Rd, Herston Qld 4006.

Craig Sinclair Bed (Sec) MPPM. Head, Prevention Division, Cancer Council Victoria, 615 St Kilda Rd, Melbourne Vic. 3004.

Terry Slevin BA (Hons) MPH FPHAA. Education and Research Director, Cancer Council Western Australia, 15 Bedbrook Pl, Shenton Park WA 6008.

Victoria Snaidr BBioMedSc MBBS (Hons). Research Fellow, Skin and Cancer Foundation Inc., University of Melbourne, 80 Drummond St, Carlton Vic. 3053.

Jamie von Nida MB BS FACD. Consultant Dermatologist, Sir Charles Gairdner Hospital, Nedlands WA 6009.

David Whiteman BMedSc MBBS (Hons) PhD FAFPHM. Professor and Group Leader, Cancer Control Group, QIMR Berghofer Medical Research Institute, 300 Herston Rd, Herston Qld 4006.

Introduction

Terry Slevin

We all spend time in the sun and we all want a healthy life. If these two things are true for you, then this book is important to you. And chances are, as you've bothered opening its pages, you or someone close to you has had skin cancer.

That is not an uncommon thing in Australia or New Zealand. In fact, it's so common that skin cancer is known by some in the cancer world as 'the Australian cancer'.

We live in a sunny place – and we revel in that. A week cannot go by without us hearing about the sun – we get too much or we get too little, skin cancer, eye problems, vitamin D problems. Despite all that, most of us are happy to read a weather forecast that predicts a sunny day.

This book is about understanding how to get the very best out of our sunny climate, while minimising the risk that is inherent in it.

A little history

Put simply, Australia and New Zealand are countries now made up of people who mostly do not have a skin type that suits our climate. Indigenous people of our islands are naturally darker skinned. Recently scientists have postulated that this is Darwinism on display. Family lines of pale skinned people did not survive as long in the intensive sun we experience, compared to people with darker or 'pigmented' skin.

People who evolved in our lands over thousands of years developed dark skin to protect themselves from that sun. The further north they went, the closer they got to the equator, the more they were exposed to the sun, the darker their skin colour became.

Then a few hundred years ago a great immigration occurred, in the form of European settlement. It led to more people living here with skin types better suited to northern Europe. For the first one and a half centuries of European settlement those people retained much of their social norms of covering up with clothing and hats, as they would have in the lands from which they came.

More recently, social norms have changed. Displaying more skin in public is not only acceptable, it has become standard. It also symbolises the free and easy outdoor lifestyle we love and cherish.

But for that 'freedom' we pay a price. And that price is skin cancer. And a high price it is.

The cost of skin cancer

Recent projections suggest we are likely to see close to a million (yes, 1 000 000) skin cancers treated per year in Australia before the end of this decade. They will range from some fairly low-impact basal cell carcinomas (BCCs) that might be quite easily treated with a topical cream which causes no more than inconvenience and discomfort for a few weeks, through to aggressive advanced melanoma, which might cause death within a few short months of diagnosis.

Non-melanoma skin cancers (NMSCs) make up most of the skin cancers: about 11 000 melanomas are currently diagnosed in Australia each year. NMSCs are so common they are not counted by our cancer registries, so much of our data on these are estimates. But the numbers are doubtless enormous. And every single one generates anxiety, often a scar and all too often far more serious impacts.

Add to the health and human cost the financial cost. When we include the out-of pocket-expenses of all the people who have skin cancers removed, to the cost to the health care system, lost productivity and other costs, by 2020 the cost per year in Australia could be approaching $1 billion.

No matter how it is measured, Australia and New Zealand are far and away the skin cancer champions of the world. And we are still to come to terms with how to cope with the extremes of sun exposure (ultraviolet radiation, UV or UVR) that reaches us for a large part of our lives.

A family issue

If you are among the hundreds of thousands, probably well over a million Aussies or Kiwis alive today who has had a skin cancer removed, then it is also likely that your skin colour has been passed to your kids and they will pass it to theirs. And that makes them vulnerable to skin cancer in the same way you were. And that makes skin cancer a family issue.

So if you've come this far you'll know that you and your family, we, all of us, need to learn more of the complexities of this disease and, perhaps most importantly, understand some of the complexities of how to prevent it. Frustratingly, it is not as simple as it seems.

Why a book?

With that in mind, this book aims to bring together some of the country's and in some cases the world's leading experts in various aspects important to the sun, health and skin cancer – prevention, diagnosis or treatment and what happens after.

Each author has a different perspective.

Some have dedicated their professional lives to treating the disease, some to researching various aspects of importance to its cause, or its prevention. Those experts tackle the mysteries of skin cancer, its various forms and what evidence we have on its causes, on UV radiation and the curious world of the solarium (albeit with its limited future in Australia). They fill us in on sunscreens and shade and their strengths and weaknesses as tools for sun protection. They walk us through how tanning happens and how it came to be a behaviour we indulge in. They cover eye health and the impact of UVR on our eyes. Of course the controversies about vitamin D could not be ignored, so a chapter on what we do and don't know about vitamin D is key.

There are also chapters that deepen our understanding of how to spot, manage and recover from skin cancer.

Some of our experts bring a very personal perspective, and that's OK. All know their stuff and all use their experience and passion to explain their field.

And all would like to know more. There is no doubt we do not have all the answers when it comes to the sun, health and skin cancer. There remain many unknowns about treating advanced disease. We do not have a system for identifying, with 100% accuracy, the dangerous skin cancer from the harmless skin spot. There are numerous debates about the precise causal pathways. And of course there are many, many controversies. Questions abound on vitamin D (have we gone too far and are now suffering more from too little sun?), nanoparticles in sunscreen, sunscreen effectiveness, methods of detection, solarium bans and more.

Each and every fact and issue raised here can be found – somewhere or other – on the web. We all have it at our fingertips. What this book does is bring the most relevant and up to date information of relevance to skin cancer into one place. It is a fast and easy reference that gives access to the best information science can currently muster, to answer important skin cancer questions.

By the time it is published, some of it will be out of date. That is the nature of a field where constant research is underway. New theories, new cures, new evidence will emerge to challenge what is on these pages. That is a good thing.

Personal note – why bother doing this?

I have worked in skin cancer prevention for 20 years.

In that time I have seen an enormous change in our acceptance of its importance, the level of understanding of skin cancer issues in the community and what we can do about it.

I have also seen confusion, misinformation and misunderstanding, and I've been frustrated with the lack of commitment and investment in prevention as a means of reducing the burden skin cancer has on the people around me.

I have my own story. Of Anglo-Celtic stock, I grew up in the 1960s and 1970s when back-slapping your mates in the school playground on Monday morning was the way to find out who had been to the beach that weekend. Busting blisters onto the inside of school shirts was considered a bonus and a red peeling nose was a sign that summer had arrived.

After having worked at the Cancer Council for about 10 years I had my own brush with skin cancers to deal with. A handful of BCCs on the face and a deeper one on the left shoulder was a remnant of my sun-soaked youth in the coastal city of Newcastle.

I recall first seeing the first Sid Seagull 'Slip Slop Slap' adverts on telly when I was in my late teens. So my generation is the last to have spent a childhood not knowing about sun protection and skin cancer.

There are signs that those early efforts, exhorting us to 'Slip on a shirt, Slop on some sunscreen and Slap on a hat' might actually be starting to influence the skin cancer statistics. It takes between 20 and 40 years for cancer prevention efforts to really take effect.

And those efforts need to be widespread.

I have to stop myself approaching sunbathing teens on the beach, or tapping the shoulder of the bloke who is putting sunscreen on just before jumping in the pool (it is likely to wash off). When in the pool, swimming laps, I want to point out to the woman wearing the rashie that the UV at 5.30 p.m. is not going to do her damage. While in a supermarket checkout queue, I want to tell the bloke in front that maybe the GP should look at that spot on his neck.

I can't help feeling that a better understanding of the basics, like:

- how skin cancer works
- how the UV levels fluctuate throughout the day and throughout the year
- how sunscreen functions
- the role shade can play in our homes, public buildings, workplaces and schools
- how to keep an eye out for early signs for skin cancer
- what to expect if they do come along.

… will serve us all better.

I hope this book sits in family bookcases, finds its way into Christmas stockings and is sitting on the pillow when people arrive home from day surgery after another round of skin cancer treatment. I hope families talk about its content. I hope they debate its precision, or whether something has been reported in the news that might make something in these pages obsolete.

Most of all, I hope people flick through its pages and learn something about skin cancer and then do something about it.

Who is it for?

This book is important to those who have had skin cancer and want to reduce their chance of getting more. It is not too late to start covering up!

But perhaps more importantly, this book aims to give information to families. Families who want to pass on the knowledge and tips for skin cancer prevention, based on sound science, to their kids and to their extended families, so that we can tackle and face one of the most preventable of cancers. Ultimately we want the antipodeans to step off the dais of skin cancer champions. We want to join the ranks of countries where skin cancer is more an oddity that does not dominate the cancer statistics.

Particularly the men

I take this opportunity to lean on the blokes. It drives me nuts that the rates of skin cancer in Australia have been going up for 30 years, but the rates in men are increasing alarmingly fast. Much more than for women. It is now the case that men are about twice as likely to be diagnosed with skin cancer as are women and that, when diagnosed, men are about twice as likely to die of the disease. There seems no biologically plausible reason for this. Rates of melanoma were similar in men and women in the early 1980s when accurate records began in Australia.

Our culture seems to create an expectation that women will care for their skin and their appearance far more than seems the norm for men. It must be time to turn this around. Ladies, please, if the blokes in your lives are not getting on board, weigh into them!

Maybe we can reduce this disease to a minor and easily managed condition taking far fewer of our resources, and of course far fewer lives. We have come some of the way, but there is still a bit of work to do before we get to that point.

Chapter 1

What is skin cancer and how does it form?

David Whiteman and Catherine Olsen

Key messages

- Australia and New Zealand experience by far the highest rates of skin cancer in the world.
- Excessive sun exposure is the most likely cause of the large majority of skin cancers, so the majority of skin cancer is preventable.
- Keratinocyte cancers (abbreviated here as KCs, and also commonly referred to as non-melanoma skin cancers or NMSCs), are by far the most common form of skin cancer.
- Melanomas are less common than KCs, but are responsible for the most deaths from skin cancer.
- People with lighter skin colours are at higher risk of skin cancer compared to people with darker skin colours.
- Family history influences skin colour and plays a major role in determining who is at higher risk of skin cancer.
- People with a past history of BCC and SCC have about a three-fold higher risk of developing melanoma than the population average.

Apples and oranges: the different types of skin cancer

What is the skin, exactly?

The skin is the largest organ in the body, and performs many different functions. The skin is our outermost protective barrier – its job is to keep out germs, toxins, radiation and a host of other nasties in the environment. The skin also regulates our temperature – keeping us warm in winter and cool in summer. To perform its many functions, the skin is made up of different types of cells in different layers (see Fig. 1.1). The outermost layer is called the epidermis, and it mostly contains flat cells called keratinocytes. It is these cells, the keratinocytes, that dry out to form the flaky outermost layer of keratin. Keratin is also used to form hair and nails. Another common cell found in the epidermis is the pigment cell or melanocyte, so called because it produces melanin. Melanin is the compound that tans our skin and gives freckles and hair their distinctive colours. Other cells found in the epidermis include sensory cells and immune cells.

The next layer down is the dermis, which contains fat, nerves, blood vessels and the bundles of fibres which give the skin its strength and flexibility. Below the dermis are the deeper fat layers. Between the epidermis and dermis is a very thin membrane, which forms a very important landmark for describing skin cancer. Cancers that are contained wholly within the epidermis and which have not crossed the boundary into the dermis, are considered pre-invasive cancers. That is, they are cancers that have not yet invaded into the deeper layers of the skin. Such cancers are

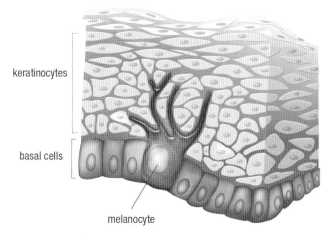

Fig. 1.1: The epidermis as viewed under a microscope. ©QIMR Berghofer Medical Research Institute.

considered to be very early stage cancers. Their technical name in Latin is *in situ*, which means literally 'in position' or 'in its natural place'. In contrast, invasive skin cancers are those which have spread from the epidermis and crossed the boundary into the dermis.

Cell division

As we go about our lives, we are constantly shedding skin cells. Each and every day, we scrape and scratch and damage our skin. To replace the cells that are being lost and to prevent our skin from being worn away completely, the skin cells undergo an orderly process of cell division (which scientists call 'mitosis'). In this process, a 'mother' cell in the lowest layer of the epidermis divides into two 'daughter' cells. Each daughter cell is an exact copy of the mother cell and contains all of the genetic material that is needed to function as a skin cell. The process of cell division is under extremely tight control to make sure that each new cell is a perfect copy of the original. This control also makes sure that cells divide only when they are supposed to. Sometimes, however, the genetic material inside a cell is damaged, for example by exposure to ultraviolet radiation in sunlight or by infection with a virus. These types of events can mutate (or disrupt) the genes inside the cell. Because each daughter cell is an exact copy of the mother cell, a mutation that occurs in a gene in the mother cell will be passed on to the daughter cells (Fig. 1.2). Many mutations have no bad effects, and some mutations can even have good effects. However, if a mutation occurs in one of a very small number of genes that are critically important for mitosis, then it can have very bad effects. For example, some mutations can make a cell keep dividing when it is not supposed to,

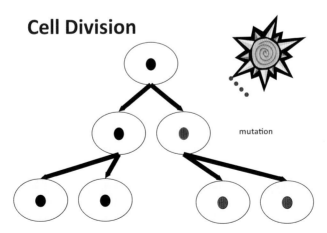

Fig. 1.2: The process of cell division. Here, one of the daughter cells has developed a mutation as a result of high-energy wavelengths of sunlight. This mutation is then passed on to the next generation of daughter cells.

leading to uncontrolled, continuous cell division. This type of uncontrolled behaviour is the classic feature of cancer. This is why cancers are sometimes called 'growths' – quite literally, the relentlessly dividing mass of cells leads to a big lump of growing tissue.

Cancers of the skin

Any of the cells that are found in the skin can, at least in theory, form cancers. By far the most common cancers are those that arise from the keratinocytes. Keratinocyte cancers occur as two main types called basal cell carcinoma (BCC) and squamous cell carcinoma (SCC). These two types of skin cancer earn their names because of how they appear when viewed under a microscope.

BCCs are the most common of all cancers in humans. They typically occur from the middle decades of life, and become more frequent with age. While most common on the face, scalp and neck, they also occur on the trunk and limbs. These cancers are often first noticed as a lump or sore on the skin that does not heal. Another name for BCCs is 'rodent ulcer'. This name describes their appearance (i.e. an ulcer on the skin usually with rolled edges), as well as their tendency to burrow into the skin. Fortunately, most BCCs grow quite slowly and can be treated very effectively.

SCCs are the second most common cancers in humans. They tend to occur on parts of the body that get lots of sun, such as the face, ears, neck, scalp and arms. They are very rare on body parts that are not exposed to the sun. Like BCCs, they often come to attention as a skin sore, but they tend to grow more quickly than BCCs. In rare cases, they can invade the bloodstream and spread through the body. For this reason, it is important to treat them early.

Melanomas are cancers that arise from the pigment cells of the skin. These cancers usually come to attention as a 'funny mole' on the skin. They are noticed most often because they have changed in colour or shape or feel. While melanomas are often dark in colour, some can be light-coloured and so can be difficult to see on the skin. Melanomas can arise anywhere on the body but the greatest numbers occur on the back; many also arise on the legs, arms and head. Melanomas can grow and spread to other parts of the body very quickly, so it is important to diagnose them early.

Other types of skin cancer include Merkel cell carcinoma, Kaposi's sarcoma, various lymphomas and other rare types. Merkel cell carcinoma is a rare but highly aggressive skin cancer, which forms from Merkel cells. Merkel cells are also found in the epidemis of the skin. It was recently discovered that most of these cancers appear to be caused by a virus (the so-called 'Merkel cell polyomavirus').

Merkel cell tumours can be flesh-coloured, pink or blue, and usually present as firm painless nodules.

Kaposi's sarcoma (KS) is a tumour that used to be very rare but became much more common during the 1980s with the HIV/AIDS epidemic. Unlike the other cancers of the skin, Kaposi's sarcoma does not arise from keratinocytes or melanocytes in the epidermis, but from the cells that line lymph or blood vessels.

The abnormal cells of KS form purple, red or brown blotches or tumours on the skin. Interestingly, these cancers are also caused by a virus, in this case, the human herpes virus 8 (HHV8). This virus is reasonably common and actually does not harm people, unless their immune system has been damaged (e.g. following infection with HIV).

Why all the fuss? The burden of skin cancer

Skin cancers impose a massive toll on the Australian population. Indeed, it is hard to overstate the burden from these diseases. The bald statistics make for sober reading. Each year, more than 400 000 Australians develop at least one BCC or SCC – that's more than 1000 people every single day of the year. Skin cancers are so common that they account for more than 80% of all cancers diagnosed in Australia. They impose the highest costs on the Australian health system of any cancer type. More than 750 000 treatments for skin cancer are billed through Medicare each year, costing the Australian government more than half a billion dollars. (These costs do not include the very large out-of-pocket expenses to patients that add to the total bill, such as gap payments to doctors and the costs of dressings, painkillers, time off work etc.) By 2015, the figures are predicted to rise to nearly 1 million skin cancer treatments at a cost to Medicare of $703 million. Often mistakenly thought of as trivial cancers, BCCs and SCCs cause enormous ill health and, unfortunately, kill many more people than we might realise. Each year in Australia, BCCs and SCCs lead to 85 000 hospital admissions (more than twice the number of admissions for each of bowel, breast or prostate cancers) and cause 500 deaths. BCCs are rarely fatal; most deaths from keratinocyte cancers are due to SCCs.

Melanomas add to this terrible burden. In 2012, more than 200 Australians every week were diagnosed with these dangerous skin cancers, resulting in an annual total of more than 11 000 people with new melanomas. Not counting BCC and SCC, melanoma is the third most commonly occurring cancer in Australian men (after prostate and bowel cancers) and women (after breast and bowel cancers). The rate at which Australians develop melanoma is the highest in the world.

Each year, out of every 100 000 people living in this country, 57 will be newly diagnosed with melanoma. This is much higher than the rate of melanoma observed in other western countries such as the USA, UK, Canada and Sweden. Only our nearest neighbour, New Zealand, has a rate of melanoma approaching that of Australia, affecting ~41 people out of every 100 000.

Melanoma has a higher death toll than other types of skin cancer. Each year, more than 1500 Australians die from this disease, making melanoma deaths more common than road fatalities.

Trends over time

Many health systems (including every state in Australia) maintain registries which are notified whenever a person living in a particular region is diagnosed with cancer. Such cancer registries are very important for monitoring trends in cancer occurrence, as well as to assess patterns of care, treatment services and cancer survival. While cancer registries aim to capture information on every diagnosis, the fact is that only a very small number of registries anywhere in the world record information about BCC and SCC (this is because BCC and SCC are three to four times more common than all other cancers combined, and collecting information on them would use up all the resources of a cancer registry). In Australia, it has been possible to monitor trends in BCC and SCC through analysis of Medicare records (Medicare is the universal health insurance which reimburses doctors for the costs of treating patients). Medicare makes payments depending upon the size of the skin cancer, its location on the body and the complexity of treatment required. A very recent analysis has shown that while treatment rates for BCC and SCC continue to climb rapidly among older Australians, the numbers of treatments for skin cancer among younger Australians (under 45 years) are beginning to fall (see Fig. 1.3). It is thought that these declines may reflect the impact of sun protection campaigns which commenced in the 1980s.

All cancer registries record diagnoses of melanoma and it is true to say that, almost without exception, melanoma rates have been rising in all populations with European ancestry (Fig. 1.4). Depending on the population, some have observed differences by sex (e.g. increased rates in men rather than women), by body site (e.g. rapid increases on the back and trunk in some regions, but not in others), or in particular age groups (particularly in older men). Monitoring such trends is extremely important to identifying shifts in the patterns of skin cancer, so that doctors and health workers can target resources to those at highest risk.

An important observation is that deaths from melanoma have not risen nearly as rapidly as diagnoses of melanoma. For example, in the USA, diagnoses of melanoma increased about

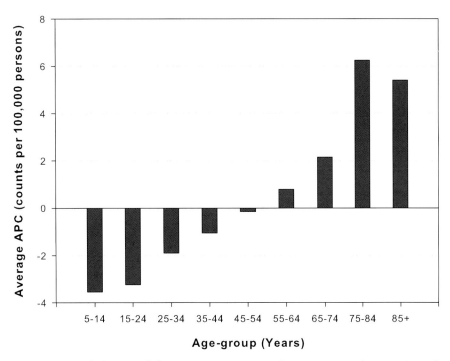

Fig. 1.3: Average rate of change of skin cancer treatments by age group. Source: Data from Medicare Australia 2000–2011.

five-fold between 1950 and 1990, whereas melanoma deaths increased only slightly less than two-fold during the same period. Similar observations have been made in western and northern Europe. In Australia, the most recent data suggest that deaths from melanoma remained stable between 1989 and 2002 for men, and declined for women (-0.8% p.a.). When looking at melanoma death rates by age group, it was found that rates were lower among people aged less than 54 years and were static among those aged 55–79 years, but continued to rise among those aged 80 years and older.

Another notable feature of recent melanoma trends around the world has been the rapid rise in the incidence of *in situ*, thin and early stage melanomas. Such increases have led some to suggest that the recent increase in melanoma may be due to overdiagnosis – that is, skin lesions are now being called 'melanomas' that would have been called 'funny moles', or not diagnosed, in the past. There are arguments for and against this notion, but most researchers agree that even if there has been some overdiagnosis of melanoma, it does not account for all the increase that has been seen during the past few decades.

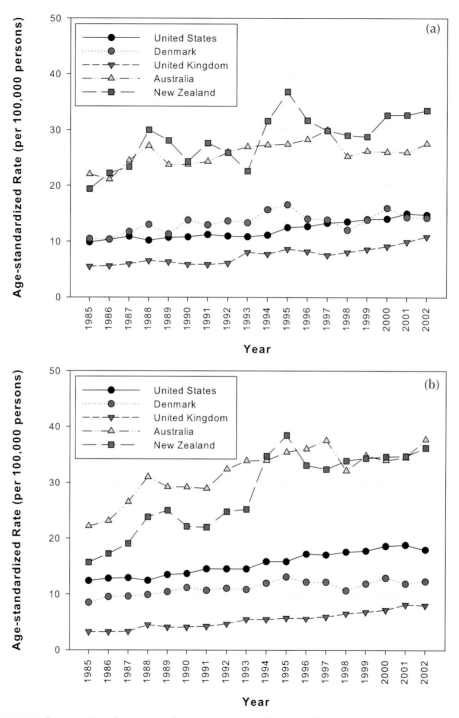

Fig. 1.4: (a) Melanoma incidence trends over time in white populations – females. (b) Melanoma incidence trends over time in white populations – males. Source: Data from Ferlay *et al.* (2010).

Who gets skin cancer?

BCCs, SCCs and melanoma are overwhelmingly cancers of fair-skinned people – especially those who trace their ancestry to northern Europe. While cancers of the skin do occur among non-European peoples, they do so at a much lower rate than among Europeans. The clearest evidence for this is when we compare the rates of skin cancer among people of different ancestry who live in the same location. For example, in the USA and New Zealand, melanoma rates are up to 10 times higher among fair-skinned residents with European ancestry (recorded by the respective health systems as 'non-hispanic Whites' in the USA and 'Pakeha' in New Zealand) than among those with non-European ancestry (e.g. 'Hispanics' and 'Blacks' in the USA, 'Maori' in New Zealand).

Skin cancer rates also vary enormously depending upon where people live. Among people with fair skin, rates of skin cancer tend to be higher among those who live in tropical or subtropical regions close to the equator (i.e. at low latitudes) than among those living in temperate or colder regions further from the equator. This was first observed back in the 1950s by Australian statistician Herbert Lancaster, who described the 'latitude gradient' for melanoma. Thus, the highest melanoma rates are seen among the predominantly European populations of Australia. Even within Australia, residents of tropical Queensland have higher melanoma rates (65 melanomas per 100 000 people per year) than those residing in New South Wales (47 melanomas per 100 000 people per year) or Victoria (36 melanomas per 100 000 people per year). After Australia, the next highest melanoma rates are seen in the white populations of New Zealand, South Africa and the USA. Much lower melanoma rates are seen in most countries in Europe. In Africa, Asia, the Pacific Islands and large parts of South America – populations with mostly non-European ancestry – rates of skin cancer are very low (Figs 1.5, 1.6).

Unlike most other parts of the world, skin cancer rates in Europe do not follow the latitude gradient described above. The highest melanoma rates in Europe are actually seen in the high-latitude countries of Scandinavia, while the lowest rates are seen in the nations of southern Europe around the Mediterranean. At first, this might seem like a paradox – if sunlight causes melanomas, and southern Europe has more sunlight than northern Europe, then southern Europe should have more melanomas than northern Europe.

However, the melanoma burden in Scandinavia is blamed on a 'perfect storm' of forces that have combined to produce high rates of melanoma. These forces include a susceptible population (i.e. mostly fair-skinned, blond-haired, blue-eyed people), coupled with the strong social desirability of a tan, the widespread use of tanning lamps and a huge increase in cheap flights to sunny holiday locations. For all these reasons, the countries of Scandinavia now have the highest rates

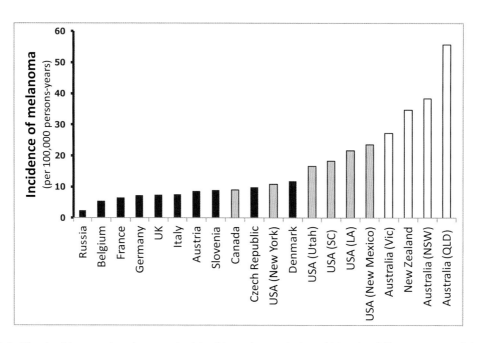

Fig. 1.5: The incidence of melanoma in fair-skinned populations living in different parts of the world. Blue bars = Europe, purple bars = North America, yellow bars = Oceania.

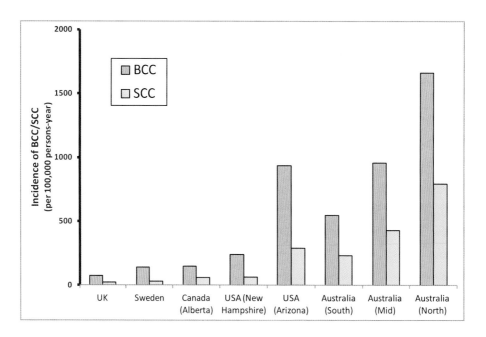

Fig. 1.6: The incidence of BCC and SCC in fair-skinned populations living in different parts of the world.

of melanoma in Europe. In contrast, the peoples of southern Europe, although exposed to much more sunshine than those in northern Europe, have darker complexions (e.g. olive skin, brown or black hair, brown eyes) which make them much less susceptible to melanomas and keratinocyte cancers. These risk factors will be discussed below, but for now they explain why the skin cancer rates in some countries are not always what we expect based on geography alone.

Skin cancer at different ages

All cancers are rare before the age of 60 years. Even so, cancers do occur in younger people, and skin cancers are no exception. Indeed, many people are surprised to learn that melanoma is by far the most common cancer occurring in young Australian adults. In 2009, there were 5469 cancers diagnosed in men and women aged 20–39 years; more than 1200 of these were melanomas (i.e. 23% of all cancers in this age group). After age 40, the rate of melanoma climbs steadily and peaks around age 80. However, the melanoma rates do not increase to the same extent on all sites of the body. In all countries, melanomas become more and more common with advancing age on body sites that are exposed to the sun (face, ears, head and neck). In contrast, melanoma rates on the back and chest tend to peak around 60 years, then become less common with age. The reasons for these differences are not well understood, but they may reflect the very different patterns of sun exposure at different body sites. Another possibility is that the pigment cells (melanocytes) on the head have a higher threshold for becoming cancerous compared to melanocytes on the trunk, and this means they are more likely to occur in later life. Scientists are attempting to resolve these complex issues now.

BCCs and SCCs are both rare in people aged less than 40 years, but start to become much more common as people pass through their 50s, 60s and 70s. It is estimated that more than one in three Australians will develop an SCC or BCC by age 70.

Skin cancer in men and women

Men and women get skin cancer at different rates. In Australia, as far back as records have been kept, men have always developed more melanomas than women. Rates were very similar in the early 1980s but since then the rate of growth of melanoma in men has been much higher in Australia than the rate of growth in women. In other countries, however, it has been women who have suffered a higher burden of melanoma. For example, in the past, New Zealand women were slightly more likely to develop melanomas than men, but recent increases in melanoma rates in young men have resulted in similar rates for men and women. Similar patterns have been observed in other countries where melanoma is not so common. In Scotland, for example, women have always developed melanoma about twice as commonly as men but, as has happened in New Zealand, rates in men have increased recently so that the rates in men and women are now about the same.

Skin cancers on different body sites

Each of the main types of skin cancer occurs at different rates on different parts of the body. For example, doctors have long observed that SCCs generally occur on highly sun-exposed areas – mostly the face, ears and neck, but also the arms and legs of people who have spent a lot of time in the sun. BCCs also occur mostly on the face, but a surprisingly large number occur on the shoulders and upper chest.

Melanomas, however, occur all over the body surface – even on the soles of the feet, inside the eye and within the lining of the gut. In strictly numerical terms, the largest numbers of melanomas are found on the back and shoulders in men, and on the legs in women. These patterns are seen in all fair-skinned populations, regardless of where in the world they are reported.

For scientists trying to understand how melanomas arise, simply comparing numbers of melanomas on a large area of the body (e.g. the back) with the numbers of melanomas arising on small area (e.g. the ear) does not really answer the question 'Is a pigment cell on the back more or less likely to turn into a melanoma than a pigment cell on the ear?' This is because large areas of skin contain more pigment cells than the ear and so, just by chance alone, a large area is likely to generate more melanomas than a small area. To get around this problem, researchers have calculated melanoma rates at different body sites taking into account their differences in surface areas. When this is done, the 'area-corrected rates' of melanoma are found to be highest on the face in both sexes, then the shoulders and back in males, and the shoulders, upper arms and back in females. Very low rates of melanoma are observed on protected sites such as the buttocks and the scalp in women.

What causes skin cancer?

All cancers, including skin cancers, arise through a series of complex steps, involving multiple factors which contribute to their development. While the precise sequence of events that cause each individual skin cancer will be unique, it is possible to identify common factors by studying the development of many thousands of skin cancers.

This is the same as saying that every single car accident is caused by a combination of unique factors, e.g. the identity and experience of the drivers, the makes of cars involved, the speed at which they were driving, the visibility, time of day, road conditions and location etc. Nonetheless, by reviewing the files of thousands of traffic accident investigations, it is possible to work out the common factors that increase the risks of having a crash.

Cancers almost always start with one or more mutations in key genes in the cells of origin (in this instance, the cells of the skin). These mutations lead to chaotic overgrowth of the affected cells. As the cancer grows, there is often some local breakdown in immune function that would normally kill diseased cells. In addition, the cancer has to develop a blood supply to nourish itself. Each of these steps is critical for the cancer to evolve, and each is made possible by different types of factors. For skin cancers, we tend to separate those factors located outside the body (i.e. the environment) from those factors inside the body (i.e. the host).

Environmental factors

Sunlight

Without question, the most potent cause of BCCs and SCCs is sunlight. There are many lines of evidence implicating sunlight as the main cause of BCC and SCC. Doctors have long known that SCCs and BCCs are found almost exclusively on sun-exposed body sites, and almost never occur on skin that is routinely shielded from the sun. Both of these cancers are especially common in outdoor workers with sun-damaged skin. Skin cancer rates are also much higher in fair-skinned people living in tropical regions than in those living in temperate regions. People born in temperate regions (e.g. the UK) who then migrate to sunny regions (e.g. Australia) as children develop BCCs and SCCs at rates that are markedly higher than if they had remained in their country of origin. Finally, SCCs can be induced in animals by exposing their skin to artificial sunlight. For all these reasons, there is no debate as to the primary role of sunlight in causing keratinocyte cancers.

Sunlight is also a major cause of melanoma, although the relationship between sunlight and melanoma is more complex than for keratinocyte cancers. Looking at the big picture, the evidence for sunlight as a cause of melanoma is strong. For example, as for BCCs and SCCs, melanomas occur more commonly in fair-skinned, sun-sensitive people, and rates of melanoma are generally highest in geographic areas receiving high levels of sunlight. Again, as for BCCs and SCCs, fair-skinned migrants from high- to low-latitude countries have a lower melanoma incidence rate than native-born residents. In addition, people with a past history of BCCs and

SCCs (and who are therefore assumed to have high levels of sun exposure) have about a three-fold higher risk of developing melanoma than the population average.

However, there are some patterns that do not fit a straightforward relationship between sun exposure and melanoma. For example, unlike BCCs and SCCs, melanomas occur most commonly on the trunk in men and limbs in women – body sites which receive considerably less sunlight than the face or ears. Melanomas almost never occur on the backs of the hands – a site with high levels of sun exposure. Studies comparing the health of workers employed in different occupations find that melanoma rates in indoor office workers are consistently higher than among outdoor occupations such as farming, construction or forestry. If sunlight does cause melanomas, then what can explain these strange patterns?

Recent research has identified several possible explanations:

- the pattern of sun exposure;
- the timing of sun exposure;
- the location of the skin cells being exposed;
- the person's genetic profile.

Many studies have reported that sunburns are a stronger risk factor for melanoma than other measures of sun exposure (e.g. time spent outdoors, or outdoor work). The theory is that sunburns reflect intense episodes of exposure to sunlight, and this type of exposure is more harmful to pigment cells (the cells of origin for melanomas) than regular, long-term exposure. In other words, it seems that the pattern of sun exposure (intermittent, intense, burning) is linked to greater risk for melanoma, compared to continual, gradual, non-burning, which is more typically linked to SCC risk.

There is also consistent evidence that melanoma risk is related to the amount of sun exposure received in childhood rather than adulthood. That is, people exposed to large amounts of sunlight in childhood (perhaps through sunburns) have higher risks of melanoma than people who have less exposure when young. In other words, there is evidence that the timing of sun exposure (childhood *v.* adulthood) is important for melanoma. Third, a lot of recent research has suggested that pigment cells on different parts of the body might react differently to sunlight, depending upon where they are located. Specifically, it is thought that pigment cells on the back and limbs might be more sensitive to the effects of sunlight than pigment cells on the head or neck. It is suspected that pigment cells on the back and limbs can be damaged more easily after relatively modest amounts of sun exposure. In contrast, pigment cells on the face and neck might be more resistant to the damaging effects of sunlight, and will only be damaged after receiving large doses. In other words, the location of the skin cells being exposed is important for melanoma. Finally, genetic studies are attempting to identify the genes that confer higher or lower risks of melanoma. Some genes have already been identified that control how the body, particularly pigment cells, respond to sunlight. That is, a person's genetic profile is important for melanoma. So far, no one knows for sure whether any of these explanations are true. However, the evidence suggests that they are probably true. Until such time as definite proof is obtained, these explanations remain theories to be tested in ongoing scientific studies.

How does sunlight cause skin cancer?

The components of sunlight will be explored in detail in Chapter 2, but for now it is enough to say that sunlight comprises one part of the spectrum of electromagnetic radiation. It is the ultraviolet wavelengths of sunlight that reach the surface of the Earth that cause skin cancer. The ultraviolet wavelengths are further classified on the basis of their energy. Short-wavelength, high-energy ultraviolet radiation (UVR) with wavelengths of 290–320 nm are classed as ultraviolet-B (UVB) radiation, whereas lower-energy UVR with wavelengths in the 320–400 nm spectrum are called UVA radiation. These terms were coined in the early days of research to separate the 'burning' wavelengths of UVB from the so-called 'ageing' wavelengths of UVA.

Every time we go into sunlight, our skin cells are damaged by UV radiation. It has been shown that exposing the skin of humans and animals to even small doses of UVB causes a very particular type of damage to DNA, the genetic material of cells, which is not caused by any other agent. When viewed under a microscope, scientists can easily see the damage affecting many skin cells, using special stains that are specific for UVR mutations. Fortunately, our bodies have evolved very rapid repair systems that can recognise and cut out damaged DNA, then replace it with intact DNA. Another response to damage from UVR exposure is to increase the amount of pigment produced in the skin. This increase in pigment is what shows up in the skin as a tan. This is the body's delayed response to damage, and is basically a way of preparing the body for further damaging exposures to sunlight. It is far from a perfect sunscreen, however, and has only limited capacity to protect the cells from damage. Quite often the body's DNA repair systems fail, and the damaged sections of DNA are not replaced. If damage occurs within a critical gene, then the process of cancer can start. This event is called 'initiation'.

Artificial sources of UVR

Sunlight is not the only source of UVR to which humans are exposed. Because the body's response to UVR damage includes tanning and many people find tanned skin desirable, many people intentionally expose themselves to artificial sources of UVR for the purpose of developing a tan. Artificial sources of UVR include tanning beds or solaria. These sources of exposure will be discussed further in Chapter 3. There is strong evidence that people who use tanning devices (sunbeds, solariums, tanning beds) regularly have substantially higher risks of melanoma, SCC and BCC than people who have never used such devices. The increased risk is higher when the first use of these devices occurs before the age of 35 years. Each additional session of sunbed use per year increases the risk of melanoma by ~1.8%. Long-term use of UV lamps to treat psoriasis and other skin conditions has also been shown to increase the risk of developing melanoma.

Probably the most powerful example of the hazards of tanning beds is demonstrated by recent events in the north Atlantic island nation of Iceland. Historically, the population of Iceland had very low rates of melanoma, as might be expected given the low levels of sunlight and cold climate of this sub-Arctic environment. Beginning around 1950, melanoma rates in Iceland began to climb at a slow but steady rate, increasing at the rate of ~2% per year. But then something quite unexpected happened. Suddenly, in the early 1990s, melanoma rates began to rise rapidly. The interesting thing was that melanoma rates increased only among women (~12% per year). The increase was most marked among younger women, and was particularly noticeable for melanomas occurring on the trunk (increasing at ~20% per year). Looking for possible explanations for the increase in melanoma rates, investigators focused on the role of sunbeds. It was noted that in 1979 there were only three tanning salons in the whole of Iceland. By 1988, the small population of Iceland (less than 250 000 people) was serviced by 56 tanning salons offering their clients more than 200 sun beds. Business was booming. Surveys showed that these facilities were heavily used by the local population; one survey conducted in 2001 found that among Icelanders aged 20–39 years, 16% of women and 12% of men had used a sun bed more than 100 times. The latest figures suggest that the situation is now improving, with melanoma rates beginning to fall since sunbeds became more heavily regulated in Iceland. However, other countries in northern Europe, notably Sweden, have also seen steady increases in melanoma incidence in recent decades, which may also be attributable to widespread use of sunbeds.

Other sources of radiation

Humans are exposed to other forms of radiation besides sunlight. The only wavelengths of radiation (besides UVR) that have been linked to cancers are the ionising wavelengths – i.e. the high-energy X-rays, gamma rays and other short wavelengths used for medical, scientific, industrial or military applications. The earliest reports that ionising radiation might lead to skin cancer were published in the 1800s, when it was noticed that radiation workers developed skin cancers on their hands. Follow-up of survivors from the atomic bomb blasts in Japan following World War 2 found higher than expected rates of BCCs in people exposed to radiation. These types of observations led to very strict controls regulating exposures to radiation in the workplace. These days, the most likely source of radiation exposure in everyday life is through medical applications, like CT scans.

Radiation therapy is a common form of treatment for certain types of cancers. This treatment involves targeting high-energy X-rays or other forms of radiation on cancers growing inside the body, to kill those that might be impossible to treat by surgery. While radiation therapy has definite benefits in terms of treating cancer, unfortunately it does have side effects. One is that the treatment can cause mutations that might lead to new cancers developing, although this occurs at very low rates. Several studies have found that keratinocyte cancers are about twice as common in people who have received radiation therapy as in people who have not. The studies suggest that BCCs are more likely than SCCs and, as might be expected, the cancers tend to occur most commonly in the field of skin that was exposed to radiation. People who are exposed to radiation therapy at young ages (less than 20 years old) seem to have the highest risks of developing skin cancer.

Although scientists have looked hard, radiation exposure does not appear to increase the risk of melanoma.

Infection

It has long been known that certain viruses can cause cancers. One particular family of viruses, the papilloma viruses, are very widespread in nature and infect many different animals. The human papilloma viruses (HPVs) have received much attention in recent years because they have been identified as the cause of cancers of the cervix in women. But these viruses are also known to cause warts in humans, and actually owe their name to the fact that they cause benign skin growths (literally 'papillomas') in many mammals. HPVs can be found on the skin of most people – they are exceedingly common. These viruses have evolved very specifically to live in the cells of the human skin, to the point where these viruses can mature and replicate only when the conditions in the skin cell are just right.

Several decades ago, scientists identified a very small number of families who had huge growths of warts all over their skin. Over time, researchers proved that the affected members of those families suffered a very rare genetic condition which led to a failure to mount an immune response to HPV. The condition was called epidermodysplasia verruciformis (EV). This discovery of a very specific immune defect leading to an infestation of HPV underscored the importance of the human immune system in maintaining a check on HPV in the skin. The skin of people with EV is literally infested with HPV and occasionally those HPV-infected warts turned cancerous. The question that arises is whether HPV can also cause skin cancer in people without EV.

This question has not been answered with certainty as yet, although there is mounting evidence that HPVs are likely to play some role in at least some skin cancers. At the present time, the evidence is strongest for SCC of the skin, based on several observations. First, HPV DNA and viral proteins have been found inside the cells of SCC, suggesting that the virus has played an active role within these tumours. In addition, HPVs have been found in the pre-cancerous skin lesions that later turn into SCCs, indicating that HPV infection occurs early in the development of the cancers. Second, patients who have had their immunity suppressed by medications have a rapid increase in risk of developing SCC, suggesting that loss of immunity allows the virus to flourish and promote cancer – this will be explored further below. However, despite these various pieces of evidence, most experts conclude that HPV alone is not sufficient to cause SCC of the skin – there needs to be some additional factor or factors (e.g. a genetic defect, medications etc.) that allow the virus to take hold and cause cancer. As new vaccines against HPV are developed and used in the population, it will be interesting to monitor the rates of SCC to see whether they confer any protection against the strains of HPV in the skin (which are different from the strains of HPV that cause cancer of the cervix).

There is no evidence that infection plays a role in the development of BCC or melanoma.

Immune suppression

People who have suppressed immunity have higher risks of developing all types of skin cancers than people with normal immune systems. Indeed, people who have had an organ transplant and who take immune-suppressing drugs to stop their grafts from being rejected have rates of skin cancer up to 100 times higher than the general population. There are at least three different ways in which these immune-suppressing drugs might lead to increased risks of skin cancer. First, some (but not all) of these drugs make the skin more sensitive to the effects of sunlight, and thus make it more likely that skin cancers will be induced. While this remains a possible explanation, it is unlikely to be the main way in which skin cancers arise in these people – only some immune-suppressing drugs cause sun sensitivity yet the rates of skin cancer are increased with almost all immune-suppressing drugs. Second, it is thought that the direct effect of these drugs in suppressing the immune system reduces the body's ability to defend against skin cancer. The third and most likely explanation is that immune-suppression by these drugs allows viruses that live in the cells of the skin (notably HPV) to replicate and infect many cells. It has been shown that HPV DNA is even more common in SCCs from transplant patients than from normal SCC patients.

Aside from immune-suppression due to drugs, the immune system can be damaged in other ways. Patients infected with HIV and patients with certain types of cancer (e.g. lymphomas) have specific types of immune defects which differ from the immune-suppression caused by drugs. Even so, patients with HIV and patients with lymphomas have increased risks of skin cancers including melanomas, highlighting the importance of a healthy immune system in preventing the development of skin cancer.

Diet

Diet plays an important role for cancers in many different organs, especially the organs of the digestive system. However, despite much research, there remains little in the way of firm evidence that diet influences a person's risk of skin cancer. Doctors and scientists have investigated many different foods and nutrients for potential effects on skin cancer, including fats, carotenoids, vitamins B, C and E, soy compounds, selenium and green tea. The results vary somewhat, but overall, the only dietary factor which seems to be associated with skin cancer with any consistency is fat. Specifically, diets low in fat are associated with lower risks of BCCs and SCCs. For all other factors investigated so far, there is no consistent evidence of any effect.

Diet does not appear to be associated with the occurrence of melanoma.

Arsenic

Arsenic is a naturally occurring element that is widely abundant in the environment. In some parts of the world, arsenic is found in drinking water, particularly bore water and well water. Arsenic is used to treat wood products (CCA, copper chromate arsenate) to prevent rotting. In Australia, CCA-treated wood is commonly used in building. Arsenic has historically been used in tonics and herbal medicines.

People exposed to high levels of arsenic over time have increased risks of cancer, particularly BCC of the skin. Indeed, until the 1960s, an 'asthma tonic' developed and distributed by a Brisbane pharmacist contained 1% arsenic trioxide (among other things); regular users later developed large numbers of BCCs. Reports from Singapore and Taiwan have documented high rates of BCCs among people who regularly used traditional Chinese remedies with high levels of arsenic.

Use of arsenic in industrial and medical applications is now tightly controlled, but people may still be exposed through bore water or through burning or handling CCA-treated timber.

Reproductive and hormonal factors

While patterns of melanomas and other skin cancers differ between men and women, there is no convincing evidence that reproductive factors or use of oral contraceptives or post-menopausal hormone replacement therapy contributes to melanoma risk.

Host factors

Skin colour and complexion

While sunlight is unquestionably the strongest cause of skin cancers, it has been known for a long time that the effects of sunlight are not the same for all people. Over tens of thousands of years, populations have adapted to the prevailing environmental conditions by evolving lighter or darker skin colours. Thus, among the long-established populations of equatorial regions (central Africa, southern India and Sri Lanka, Papua New Guinea and the islands of Melanesia), very dark skin colours have been selected to provide the strongest possible protection from the sun. In contrast, populations evolving in conditions of low sunlight (northern and western Europe) developed very light skin tones, most likely to maximise production of vitamin D. In mid-latitude locations (southern Europe, central and eastern Asia, North and South America), intermediate skin tones predominate.

During the last couple of centuries, very large numbers of fair-skinned people from Europe have migrated to the New World. Resettling in the sunnier climes of Australia, Africa and the Americas, these migrants have been exposed to levels of UVR for which their skins were not prepared. The result: epidemics of skin cancer. But the migrants from Europe were not all of one complexion. Whereas the Celts from Ireland and Scotland were more likely to have red hair, very fair skin and freckles, those from Spain, Italy and Greece tended to have more olive complexions. So while it is generally true to say that people with European ancestry have fair skins, there is a wide spectrum of skin colouring. This spectrum of skin colours translates into a spectrum of skin cancer risk. A classification scheme has been developed (the Fitzpatrick scale) to enable doctors and scientists to measure skin colour and compare results across studies (see Fig. 1.7).

Skin type chart

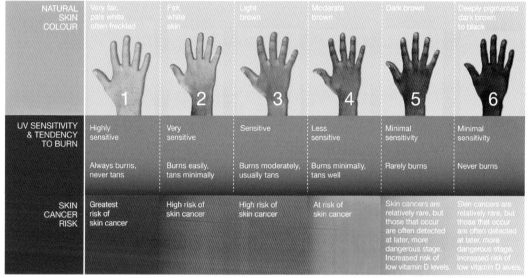

NATURAL SKIN COLOUR	Very fair, pale white, often freckled	Fair, white skin	Light brown	Moderate brown	Dark brown	Deeply pigmented dark brown to black
	1	2	3	4	5	6
UV SENSITIVITY & TENDENCY TO BURN	Highly sensitive	Very sensitive	Sensitive	Less sensitive	Minimal sensitivity	Minimal sensitivity
	Always burns, never tans	Burns easily, tans minimally	Burns moderately, usually tans	Burns minimally, tans well	Rarely burns	Never burns
SKIN CANCER RISK	Greatest risk of skin cancer	High risk of skin cancer	High risk of skin cancer	At risk of skin cancer	Skin cancers are relatively rare, but those that occur are often detected at later, more dangerous stage. Increased risk of low vitamin D levels.	Skin cancers are relatively rare, but those that occur are often detected at later, more dangerous stage. Increased risk of low vitamin D levels.

Skin Type Table adapted by SunSmart Victoria (2011) using Fitzpatrick Scale (1975). Images courtesy Cancer Research UK.

Fig. 1.7: Skin type (Fitzpatrick) classification of sun-reactive skin types. With permission of Cancer Council Victoria.

Repeated studies have found that people with fair skin that burns and does not tan (Fitzpatrick 1–2) have approximately two-fold higher risks of all types of skin cancer than people with darker skins (Fitzpatrick 4–6). Similarly, people who freckle or have light eye colour (blue/blue-grey and green) also have about a two-fold increased risk of developing BCC, SCC or melanoma when compared to people without these characteristics. Light hair colour is also associated with increased risks of melanoma and other skin cancers; the highest risks are seen with red hair, followed by blond and light brown hair. People with dark brown or black hair have the lowest risks.

Moles

Moles are small tan or brown spots which can arise anywhere on the skin surface. Moles develop during childhood and adolescence, then regress during adulthood. Children in Australia tend to develop moles more quickly than children in Europe, although it appears that the total number of moles on the skin is roughly similar regardless of location. While moles usually occur as single isolated spots, they can occur in very large numbers but with no obvious pattern. These features make them quite different from freckles, which usually occur in bunches on sun-exposed sites such as the face and arms and which tend to be more pronounced in summer and fade in winter.

Under the microscope, moles are benign growths of lots of pigment cells (melanocytes). Again, this is very different from the microscopic appearance of a freckle. A freckle occurs when one or more melanocytes produce an excess of pigment which stains the surrounding skin cells. The amount of pigment produced by the melanocytes can wax and wane, thereby changing the appearance of the freckle.

The presence of large numbers of moles ('naevi', as doctors call them) is associated with an increased risk of melanoma. This association has been shown in many studies around the world; basically, the risk of melanoma increases with the number of moles on the skin. People with more than 100 moles have up to 10 times higher risk of developing a melanoma than people with very few moles.

A common question is whether melanomas develop directly from moles, or whether moles are simply a marker that a person has a higher than average risk of developing a melanoma. As is often the case in medicine, the answer is 'Both'. It is now recognised that up to half of all melanomas grow directly from a pre-existing mole and the remainder seem to arise on their own with no prior mole.

While a very small number of studies have suggested that moles might also be a risk factor for BCCs, most studies have not found any support for this observation.

Body shape
There is some evidence that being overweight or obese may modestly increase risk of melanoma in men but not in women. Some studies have also reported that tall people have higher risks of melanoma than short people, even when we take into account the differences in body surface area. As yet, scientists do not have a good theory to explain these observations. It may be as simple as 'Big people have more skin cells, and therefore have a higher risk of one of them turning into a skin cancer', so more work needs to be done in this area.

Family history
Melanoma commonly clusters in families. People who have a first-degree (e.g. mother, father, brother, sister or child) or second-degree (e.g. grandparent, grandchild, uncle, aunt, nephew, niece, half-sibling) relative with melanoma have about double the risk of developing melanoma in their lifetime. Similarly, people whose parents have SCCs have a three-fold higher risk of SCCs than people whose parents do not have SCCs.

Genes
Ultimately, all the features that make each person unique are determined, to a greater or lesser extent, by the genes inherited from their ancestors. In recent years, there has been an explosion of

Table 1.1: Genes associated with skin cancer or risk factors

Locus	Gene	Comment	Skin cancer type
16q24	MC1R	Hair colour, freckling	BCC, SCC, melanoma
20q11	ASIP	Hair colour, freckling	BCC, SCC, melanoma
11q14	TYR	Pigmentation, freckling	BCC, SCC, melanoma
1p36	PADI6	Cytoskeletal structures	BCC
1q42	RHOU	Wnt pathway	BCC
9p21	CDKN2A	Cell cycle control	BCC, melanoma
7q32	KLF14	Transcription factor	BCC
12q13	KRT5	G138E substitution keratin protein	BCC
6p25	EXOC2	Possible pigmentation	BCC, SCC
13q32	UBAC2	Possible inflammation	BCC, SCC
5p15	TERT-CLPTM1L	Telomerase repair	BCC, melanoma

knowledge about genes. What has become clear is that the human body is under even more complex and intricate genetic control than we ever imagined. Very few processes are controlled by a single gene; it is almost always the case that whole networks of genes control each facet of the human body. We have learned that even apparently simple characteristics like hair colour, skin colour, eye colour and freckling are controlled by numerous genes. Many of these genes have been identified, but more remain to be discovered.

In spite of this complexity, much has been learned about skin cancer from small groups of patients with very rare mutations in single genes. These genes have turned out to be crucially important for skin cancer, and help us to understand how skin cancers are caused. For example, patients with a skin disease called xeroderma pigmentosum (XP) have a single mutation that renders them unable to repair DNA damaged by sunlight. Because of this, XP patients develop BCCs, SCCs and melanoma at rates up to 1000 times higher than the general population. This condition confirms the role of sunlight in causing all three main types of skin cancer.

Another example of a critically important gene mutation is epidermodysplasia verruciformis (EV). As mentioned previously, people with EV carry a mutation that prevents them from mounting an immune response to HPV infection of the skin. EV patients develop very large numbers of warts in early childhood and have very high lifetime risks of SCCs on the skin.

Despite the insights learned from these high-risk genes, most patients with skin cancer do not carry mutations in these genes. Other less dangerous but more common genes are known to play a role. Table 1.1 lists genes that have been associated either with skin cancer or risk factors. Mostly, these genes increase a person's risk of skin cancer by very modest amounts – much less than the risks associated with high levels of sun exposure. While many of the genes identified as being associated with skin cancer are also associated with complexion or moles, some interesting new genes have been discovered. It is some way off, but there is the possibility that in the future, genetic tests will be able to predict a person's risk of skin cancer.

Summary

Skin cancers are very common in Australia, and impose a huge burden on this country. It is estimated that two out of three men and one out of three women in Australia will develop a skin cancer in their lifetime. Most of these cancers will be keratinocyte or non-melanoma skin cancers (BCC, SCC), but about one in 14 Australians will develop melanoma. The risks of each type of skin cancer vary depending on the pattern, site and intensity of sun exposure. Host factors, including skin colouring and genetic factors, also affect a person's response to sunlight. Other causes of skin cancer include radiation, infections and immune suppression.

The overwhelming majority of skin cancers are caused by excessive exposure to sunlight.

Further reading

Ferlay J, Parkin DM, Curado MP, Bray F, Edwards B, Shin HR, Forman D (2010) *Cancer Incidence in Five Continents. Vols I–IX*. IARC CancerBase No. 9. International Agency for Research on Cancer, Lyon. http://ci5.iarc.fr.

Madan V, Lear JT, Szeimies RM (2010) Non-melanoma skin cancer. *Lancet* **375**, 673–685. http://www.sciencedirect.com/science/article/pii/S014067360961196X.10.1016/S0140–6736(09)61196-X.

Medicare Australia. http://www.medicareaustralia.gov.au.

Thompson JF, Scolyer RA, Kefford RF (2005) Cutaneous melanoma. *Lancet* **365**, 687–701. http://www.sciencedirect.com/science/article/pii/S0140673605179513.10.1016/S0140–6736(05)17951–3.

Whiteman DC, Whiteman CA, Green AC (2001) Childhood sun exposure as a risk factor for melanoma: a systematic review of studies. *Cancer Causes and Control* **12**, 69–82. doi:10.1023/A:1008980919928.

Whiteman DC, Pavan W, Bastian BK (2011) The melanomas: a synthesis of epidemiological, clinical, histopathological, genetic, and biological aspects, supporting distinct subtypes, causal pathways, and cells of origin. *Pigment Cell and Melanoma Research* **24**, 879–897. doi:10.1111/j.1755-148X.2011.00880.x.

Chapter 2

Ultraviolet radiation: nuts and bolts of the big skin cancer factor

Peter Gies, Stuart Henderson and Kerryn King

Key messages

- Latitudes in the Southern Hemisphere will experience 15% higher ultraviolet radiation (UVR) reaching the Earth compared to the equivalent Northern Hemisphere latitude location.
- The major factors influencing the intensity of UVR reaching the Earth's surface are the time of the day, geographic location, seasons, ozone cover, cloud cover, reflectivity of the environment, altitude, level of pollutants and the role of direct *v.* diffuse UVR.
- The UV Index is a standard and useful measure that allows us to assess the strength of the sun at any location at any time. Sun protection is recommended when the UV Index is at 3 or higher.
- There are various artificial sources of UVR, from welding machines to solaria which have potentially very high levels of UVR emission compared to some common forms of lighting which are likely to have very low levels of UVR emission.

All about the sun: UVR, ozone and the weather

Light and heat from the sun has allowed life to flourish on Earth. The sun is also a source of UVR to which the world's populations are exposed, sometimes to their detriment. The effects of these UVR exposures, or more particularly overexposures, are covered in other chapters. This chapter provides an overview of the factors that determine the levels of solar UVR at the Earth's surface and describes how the levels vary from one location to another.

In brief, the problem for Australia is we have high levels of solar UVR due to geographical location.

What we do when outdoors determines how much UVR we each receive. Use of personal protection can greatly reduce the UVR exposures and consequently the harmful effects (see Chapters 4, 5, 6, 7).

Little can or should be done to change the levels of solar UVR in any particular location. That means we need to reduce our UVR exposures and therefore, hopefully, subsequent skin cancers.

This chapter discusses UVR from the sun and the various factors that can affect the amount of solar UVR reaching the Earth's surface. How much solar UVR there is in any location is largely determined by one major thing – geographical position, in particular the latitude but also the hemisphere it is in.

Due to the Earth's elliptical orbit, it is ~1.7% closer to the sun each January when the Southern Hemisphere has its summer and a further ~1.7% from the sun in July, when the Northern Hemisphere has its summer, giving a total difference of 3.4%. Because intensity decreases substantially with increased distance, this means locations in the Southern Hemisphere receive around 7% higher solar UVR levels than equivalent places in the Northern Hemisphere.

The fact that the atmosphere in the Southern Hemisphere is less polluted than that in the Northern Hemisphere, explained largely by the smaller population in the south, also means more solar UVR is transmitted to the Earth's surface. It has been estimated that, due to the combined effect of less pollution and the Earth's orbit, locations in the Southern Hemisphere will have ~15% higher solar UVR than locations with the same latitude in the Northern Hemisphere.

Locations at the same latitude but at different longitudes can have different levels of solar UVR because one may be on the coast and another may be in the centre of a continent, e.g. Alice Springs and Brisbane in Australia. Alice Springs often has in excess of 300 sunny days a year whereas coastal regions can have more significant cloud cover and rainfall and therefore less sunshine and solar UVR.

What exactly is UVR? The ABC of UVR

Solar radiation covers the electromagnetic radiation spectrum and includes light or visible radiation in the wavelength range 400–770 nm as well as infrared and radio waves at higher wavelengths, and ultraviolet and X-rays, gamma rays and cosmic rays at lower wavelengths (see Fig. 2.1).

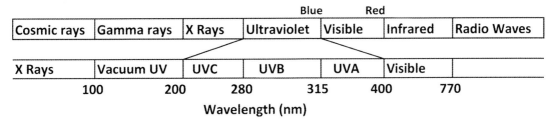

THE SPECTRUM OF ELECTROMAGNETIC RADIATION

Cosmic rays	Gamma rays	X Rays	Ultraviolet	Visible	Infrared	Radio Waves

X Rays	Vacuum UV	UVC	UVB	UVA	Visible	

100   200   280   315   400   770

Wavelength (nm)

Fig. 2.1: The spectrum of electromagnetic radiation, showing UVR between the visible and X-rays as well as where UVA, UVB and UVC fit in.

The various wavelength ranges for the ultraviolet are UVC (200–280 nm), UVB (280–315 nm) and UVA (315–400 nm) as defined by the Commission Internationale d'Eclairage (CIE, International Committee of Illumination).

First, the proportion of UVR in the sun's spectrum is actually very very small. At the top of the atmosphere, UVA makes up only ~6.8% of the total radiation from the sun and UVB makes up 1.4%, but at the Earth's surface UVA makes up 6.5% and UVB makes up 0.04% of the total radiation from the sun.

UVC is completely absorbed by the ozone layer and none reaches the Earth's surface. Below 200 nm the UVR is strongly absorbed by oxygen in the air – only wavelengths above 200 nm can affect living tissue and organisms.

UVR is strongly absorbed by human skin and tissue, generally being absorbed in the top layer of skin (~0.1–1 mm deep), with the result that the skin and the eyes will be most at risk. The shorter the wavelength, the higher the energy of the photons and the more damage they can do to the cells and molecules of the body. Therefore all UVR (UVC, UVB and UVA) photons carry more energy and have a greater potential to break chemical bonds in human and biological tissue than visible photons. Similarly, within the UVR range the shorter-wavelength, higher-energy UVC photons are more likely to cause damage than UVB photons, which in turn are considered more hazardous than UVA photons.

Seven factors affecting solar UVR

In addition to the obvious factors of geographic location, in particular proximity to the equator, and season or time of the year (both addressed in detail later), there are seven major influences affecting levels of UVR in the environment:

- solar elevation (height of the sun in the sky);
- ozone;
- cloud cover;
- ground surface reflectivity;
- the effect of altitude;
- the effects of aerosols and pollutants;
- direct and diffuse UVR.

1 Solar elevation

For clear-sky conditions, how high the sun is in the sky is the major factor that determines how much solar UVR there is. As stated previously, incoming radiation from the sun at the top of the atmosphere contains UVA, UVB and even UVC. As it passes through the atmosphere, UVA, UVB and UVC are absorbed and scattered by the atmosphere – the shorter the wavelength, the higher the scattering. UVC is completely absorbed so none reaches the Earth's surface. UVB with the next-shortest wavelengths is scattered and absorbed more than UVA, which is scattered and absorbed only slightly. Oxygen and ozone are the constituents of the atmosphere that absorb UVC and most of the UVB.

The longer the path length through the atmosphere, the more UVB is absorbed; the longest path occurs when the sun is near the horizon. This is why there is less UVR at sunrise and sunset. No matter what time of year, the UVB levels are always least hazardous when the sun is low in the sky and most hazardous when the sun is at its highest (solar noon; see Fig. 2.2). Thus the highest

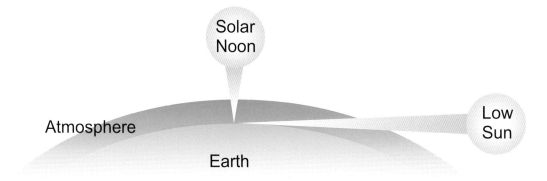

Fig. 2.2: The path length through the atmosphere is much longer when the sun is low in the sky than when it is overhead, resulting in more absorption and scattering of the shorter-wavelength UVB.

danger from the sun occurs in the middle of the day around solar noon in summer, when the sun is highest in the sky each year. When the sun is low in the sky, the path length through the atmosphere is much longer than when the sun is overhead.

Only at places within the tropics (between 23.5°N and 23.5°S) can the sun ever be directly overhead. This occurs on 21/22 December in the Southern Hemisphere, e.g. north of Rockhampton, and on 21/22 June in the Northern Hemisphere, e.g. south of Hawaii.

Thus there is a link between UV levels and temperatures as far as the seasons go, as UV Index levels are always higher in summer when it is warm, but the correlation on a day-to-day basis is much less rigorous. On clear-sky days with the same temperature, the UV Index (explained in detail later) can change from one day to the next due to changes in ozone above the location. Ozone changes naturally from day to day, sometimes by up to 40%, so two consecutive clear-sky days can have substantially different UV Indexes due solely to ozone variation.

The Earth's atmosphere is ~100 km thick. If the sun is directly overhead the path length through the atmosphere is ~100 km but, as shown in Fig. 2.2, if the sun is low in the sky the path length could be many times longer. It is twice as long when the sun is 30° above the horizon and roughly 10 times greater at sunrise or sunset. This results in much more absorption and scattering of the UVR, particularly the UVB as shorter wavelengths (UVB) are absorbed and scattered more than longer wavelengths (UVA or visible). The sun's UV energy is also spread over a larger area when the sun is low in the sky. The amount of UVB and UVA in the solar UVR is very different when the sun is low in the sky and is therefore significantly less hazardous.

The amount of solar UVR reaching the Earth on any day depends on the height of the sun in the sky and therefore changes with the seasons, with levels being greater in summer than in winter.

Figure 2.3 gives the percentage of the daily total solar UVR within certain time periods, using a specific example – the UV that reached the ground in Melbourne on 16 January 2012, a fairly typical summer day in Australia. The hours 12pm to 2pm (1 hour either side of solar noon: 1pm daylight savings time) make up 31% of the daily total, and almost 70% of the daily total occurs between the hours of 10am and 3pm DST (11am to 4pm AEST; see Table 2.1). These percentages will vary for different latitude locations and for different times of year.

2   Ozone

Ozone is a vital constituent of the Earth's atmosphere. Ozone starts absorbing UVA at ~330 nm and becomes more and more effective at absorbing UVR until by 290 nm, which is near the

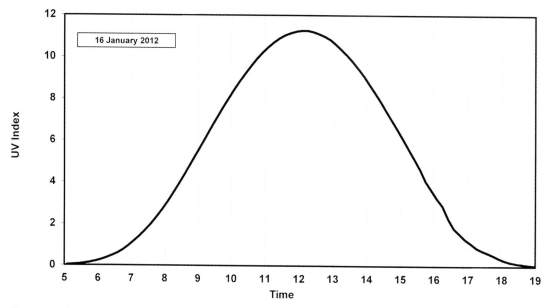

Fig. 2.3: The variation in UV Index with time of day (AEST) in Melbourne, 16 January 2012. During the hours of 10am to 3pm DST (11am to 4pm AEST) 70% of the daily total UVR is received.

bottom of the UVB part of the spectrum. Put simply, the higher the ozone, the lower the UVB and vice versa.

Since the discovery of the ozone hole over the Antarctic in the early 1980s ozone levels have been observed to decline worldwide, resulting in increased levels of solar UVR at the Earth's surface. The impacts of ozone depletion on UVR levels are most apparent in the Antarctic beneath the ozone hole, but other cases of localised depletion of ozone at mid-latitudes have been reported at numerous places around the world with subsequent increases in solar UVR.

The first evidence that ozone depletion could affect population centres was recorded in 1988 when a mass of ozone-depleted air from the break-up of the ozone hole moved north and raised the levels of solar UVR in Melbourne for over a month. Most recently, in August 2011 (winter) a large mass of air with low ozone moved down from the tropics over southern Australia. The weather was clear and sunny: record levels of solar UVR were recorded for that time of year in Perth, Adelaide, Melbourne, Canberra, Sydney and Hobart, with UV Index values up to 40% higher than normal. At the time, a study was underway on UVR exposures of outdoor workers in

Table 2.1: Daily total UVR during each hour (%)

Time	%
6–7am DST (7–8am AEST)	0.5
7–8am DST (8–9am AEST)	2
8–9am DST (9–10am AEST)	5
9–10am DST (10–11 AEST)	8
10–11am DST (11am–12pm AEST)	12
11am–12pm DST (12–1pm AEST)	15
12–1pm DST (1–2pm AEST)	16
1–2pm DST (2–3pm AEST)	15
2–3pm DST (3–4pm AEST)	12
3–4pm DST (4–5pm AEST)	8
4–5pm DST (5–6pm AEST)	4
5–6pm DST (6–7pm AEST)	1

and around Melbourne. In late August that year workers received substantial doses of UVR, significantly higher than the doses measured in early August.

Figure 2.4 shows the different UV Index readings measured in Melbourne during the study. Given the cities involved have a combined population greater than 10 million, there would have been many people who were overexposed and developed sunburn, with subsequent potential impact on skin cancer rates years later. Several scientific papers have reported measuring events of decreased ozone and simultaneous increases in solar UVR levels in Europe as well as in the Southern Hemisphere.

A recent study has estimated that, by slowing or halting the decline in ozone levels, the Montreal Protocol has helped reduce skin cancer worldwide. The Montreal Protocol was the 1987 international agreement designed to halt ozone depletion and allow the ozone layer to regenerate. The study estimated that the implementation of the Montreal Protocol will result in 2 million fewer cases of skin cancer per year being diagnosed by 2030. That translates to ~14% fewer skin cancer cases.

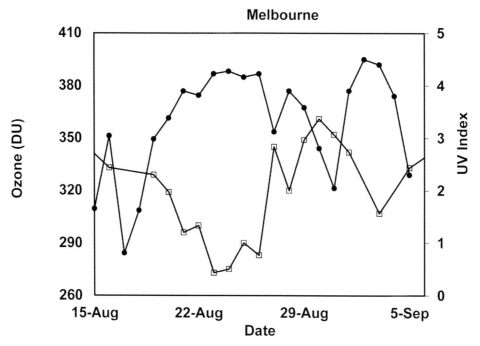

Fig. 2.4: The inverse relationship between ozone □ and UVR ● seen. Ozone □ (measured by the Bureau of Meteorology) started to decline around 19 August 2011 and the measured UV Index ● in Melbourne started to increase that same day. Source: Redrawn from Gies *et al.* (2013).

3 Cloud cover

Figure 2.5 shows the effect of clouds on the levels of solar UVR for three consecutive days in February 2009 in Sydney. As they were consecutive days, the height of the sun each day changed only very slightly and was barely perceptible. Ozone was only slightly different each of the three days, with just a small difference between 9 and 10 February (approximately a 2% difference or 5 Dobson units – the unit that is used to measure ozone). The one thing that did change noticeably was cloud cover – 8 February had fine weather and clear skies, with a measured UV Index of 12.6 and a daily total UVR of 68 SEDs (scientists have defined a standard dose of UVR as 100 Joules/square metre and called it the Standard Erythemal Dose or SED). 9 February was overcast with a resulting UV Index of 8.6 and a daily total UVR of 28 SEDs, 10 February was cloudy and overcast with some showers and a UV Index of 5.0 and 14 SEDs.

The more cloud there was, the lower were both the maximum UV Index that day and the total amount of solar UVR reaching the Earth's surface. The maximum UV Index (usually near solar noon) is an indication of the potential hazard and the daily total UVR is an indication of the

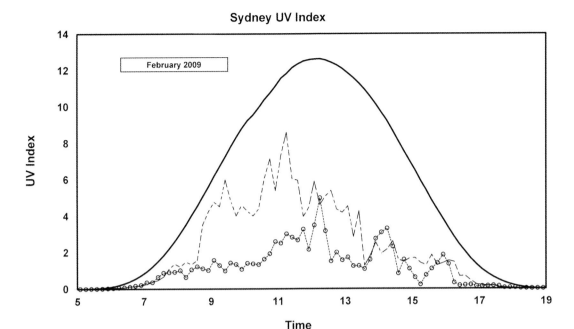

Fig. 2.5: The variation of UVR levels in Sydney, 8–10 February 2009. The height of the sun changed only slightly but weather conditions and cloud cover can change rapidly. 8 February (—) was fine weather with clear skies, 9 February (---) was mostly cloudy and 10 February (- -O- -) was overcast and rainy with UV Index levels much reduced.

maximum potential dose. Although there was significant cloud on both 8 and 9 February, the daily total UVR for those days was 28 and 14 SEDs, which is still enough for people with fair skin to be sunburned. UVB levels were reduced but not eliminated. Sometimes reflection of the sun's rays off clouds can increase UVB levels above the expected values.

4   Ground surface reflectivity

Exposures to solar UVR when outside can also depend significantly on the reflectivity (albedo) of the ground surface. While reflectivity in the UVB part of the spectrum is lower than in the visible, a highly reflective surface can increase the ambient levels of solar UVR in the vicinity. It can also cause exposure to parts of the body that are normally protected or shaded, e.g. on a sunny day at the ski fields fresh snow can have reflectivity as high as 80–90%. Many skiers have learnt the hard way and been very sunburned as well as suffering short-term eye damage due to the solar UVR reflected upwards from the snow. This gets around the body's normal defences such as eyebrows, eye sockets and eyelids. Measured reflectivity of several surfaces have been published. Surfaces like short green grass can reflect 0.8–1.6% of UVR, concrete (depending whether it is old or new) ranges from 7.0% to 15% and tar-sealed road 4.1–6.0%. The highest reflectivity levels measured were shiny corrugated iron (18% reflectivity), light dry Atlantic beach sand (15–18% reflectivity) and fresh and old snow (88% and 50% reflectivity respectively).

5   The effect of altitude

At higher altitudes solar UVR increases by ~4% for every 300 m. Measurements have shown that two locations in the European Alps, where altitudes differed by 1 km, had levels of solar UV Index that differed by 14%. The higher the altitude of a location the less chance the atmosphere has to absorb or scatter the incoming UVB radiation, so UVB levels are higher.

6   The effects of aerosols and pollutants

Aerosols are small particles suspended in the air which can attenuate or scatter solar UVR. They usually occur at altitudes below 2 km above the Earth's surface. The effect is generally less than that due to atmospheric scattering. Air pollutants in the form of gas can also absorb solar UVR but the effect is generally less than a few percent unless the levels of pollutants or dust are very high, e.g. after the eruption of Mount Pinatubo in 1991 when solar UVR was significantly reduced. Smoke from bushfires has also reduced solar UVR levels, particularly in January/February, e.g. as a result of the 2009 Black Saturday bushfires in regional Victoria.

7   Direct and diffuse UVR

What many people do not realise is that there is often more solar UVR from the sky than there is from the direct sun. In fact, for most of the day, the diffuse or scattered UVR from the sky is higher than the direct UVR from the sun (see Fig. 2.6). Only for a few hours either side of solar noon is the direct UVR greater than the diffuse. This means that if you are standing in the shade beneath a shade structure but near one edge so that you can still see large areas of the sky, the scattered UVR from those areas of sky can reach you. Over time they can cause sunburn, even though you are in the shade. This is discussed in more detail in Chapter 6.

When boating or sailing, people may get sunburned and assume it was due to reflection of solar UVR from the water. Generally this is unlikely, however, as water is highly reflective only when the sun is low in the sky and the sun's rays are at grazing incidence to the water. In this situation, the UVR is reflected but as the sun is low in the sky the damaging UVB content is very low (as is the UV Index); the effect on people will be low as well.

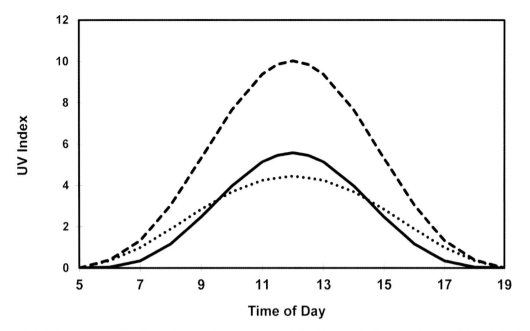

Fig. 2.6: The variation in direct (—) and diffuse (●●●●) UV Index during the day, and the global (sum of diffuse and direct) UVR in terms of UV Index (- - - -).

Sailors are often exposed to the direct sun as well as to a very large fraction of the sky. This situation is very different from that normally encountered on land, where there can often be large buildings, structures or trees within the vicinity that block diffuse solar UVR. As discussed in the previous section, the intensity of solar UVR from the sky is often higher than that from the direct sun, so sailing exposures are often due to the sum of both the large amount of diffuse solar UVR and the direct sun.

This combination of diffuse UV exposure and UV reflected from ground surfaces such as short grass and concrete explain sunburn experienced by people sitting in a shaded seat at the cricket for a day's play.

The UV Index: what does it mean and how is it useful?

Reducing exposures to solar UVR can lead to a reduction of skin cancer rates. Prevention campaigns aimed at getting the general public to reduce their exposures needed to describe the levels of UVR in a way that people could understand. A simple numerical indicator of the maximum potential solar UVR hazard each day – the UV Index – was introduced in 2002 by the World Health Organization (WHO), the World Meteorological Office (WMO), the United Nations Environment Programme (UNEP) and the International Commission on Non-Ionizing Radiation Protection (ICNIRP) (WHO 2002). The higher the number assigned to the UV Index, the higher the potential UVR hazard.

Simply put, the UV Index is the biologically effective UVR intensity multiplied by 40 to give a whole number. For example, the biologically effective or sunburning solar UVR intensity at noon in summer in Australia would be 0.3 $W.m^{-2}$ (watts per metre squared) which, multiplied by 40, gives the number 12 as the UV Index. The standardisation of solar UVR reporting allows us to compare the potential UVR hazard between different geographical locations using simple whole numbers. This can be particularly useful and important for tourists, but is also useful in communicating the UVR hazards from day to day for particular locations. The UV Index can play an important role in educational campaigns to change people's behaviour and reduce their UV exposures (Fig. 2.7).

In Australia, the Bureau of Meteorology forecasts the UV Index using computer models which incorporate various inputs such as atmospheric parameters including ozone, potential cloud cover and, to a lesser extent, water vapour and aerosols. Computer model computations work well for clear-sky solar UVR and can give an accurate estimate of the maximum UVR. With cloud cover, which can vary significantly, the forecasting of UV Index is difficult – there are more significant uncertainties for non-clear sky conditions.

To reduce the risk of overexposure to solar UVR in Australia, the state and territory Cancer Councils, the Bureau of Meteorology (BOM) and Australian Radiation Protection and Nuclear Safety Agency (ARPANSA) came up with the SunSmart UV Alert, which is issued when the UV Index is forecast to be 3 and above (Fig. 2.8). UV Alert and sun protection messages are issued if the clear-sky UV Index forecast by the BOM is 3 or greater. The UV Alert is issued to the media, newspapers, internet and smart phone apps. Originally, the UV Index was defined as the maximum value of solar UVR each day. Nowadays, with reporting of solar UVR levels live on the internet, it is used as a continuous measure. ARPANSA measures the solar UVR in the capital cities and several other major population centres and displays the data as the UV Index each minute on the ARPANSA website at http://www.arpansa.gov.au/uvindex/index.cfm

How does UVR differ across Australia?

When discussing the levels of solar UVR, there are three main measures of interest. First, the intensity or strength of the sun measured by the UV Index. Second, the total amount of time

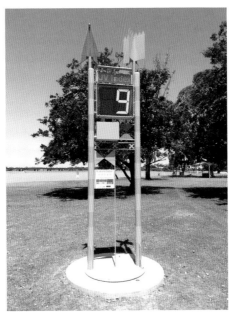

Fig. 2.7: A Live UV meter installed at Deep Water Point in Perth by the City of Melville and the Cancer Council WA. It allows people using the recreation area to judge their need for sun protection based on current UV Index levels.

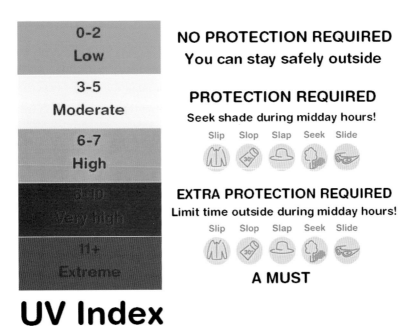

Fig. 2.8: The UV Index warning chart with cut points illustrating the levels at which the UV is considered low, moderate, high, very high and extreme, and the sun protection methods.

spent in the sun or the daily dose is important. The third factor is that different people have different skin types. Those with fair skin sunburn more easily than those with slightly darker skin. Fair-skinned people need a smaller UVR dose to get sunburn (erythema).

As described earlier, the standard dose of UVR is known as a Standard Erythemal Dose (SED). A person with skin type 2 will sunburn if they receive 2 SEDs, whereas some people with skin that can tan, e.g. skin type 3, will be sunburned at 3–4 SEDs (see Fig. 1.7, p. 21). People with darker skin may get sunburned at 8–10 SEDs. A UV Index of 12 that lasts for an hour, which is a common occurrence around Australia in summer, will deliver a dose of 10.8 SEDs, more than enough to sunburn most people.

A measure of solar UVR at different locations in Australia is usually described in terms of SEDs. The closer the location is to the equator, the higher the levels of solar UVR that reach the Earth. In summer in some parts of Australia, like a clear-sky day in Townsville, Darwin or Broome, up to 70 SEDs each day might reach the Earth. If we add the daily totals to get an annual total, the highest values will be in places nearer the equator, the lowest in places near the North and South Pole.

The annual totals follow a latitude gradient (Fig. 2.9a). However, the annual totals do not show the variability during the year. Figure 2.9b shows the variability for several cities including Darwin and Townsville in the north and Sydney and Melbourne further south. In summer there is not much difference between the two locations, but in winter Melbourne has very low levels of solar UVR (UV Index values of 2) while Townsville has UV Index values of 6 or higher (Fig. 2.10). That means that in Townsville sun protection will required year-round. The fact that the weather in Queensland is warmer also means that people wear clothing that is perhaps less protective, and continue to receive a substantial proportion of their annual UVR exposures even in winter.

UV levels around the world: similar UV levels and local circumstances

Numerous organisations, including those in New Zealand, the USA, Japan, Spain, the UK, Germany, Sweden and several locations in Norway and Finland measure solar UVR levels; these are shown in Fig. 2.11 along with levels for Australia. It is clear that the levels of solar UVR in Australia are very high – two to three times those in much of Europe, particularly Northern Europe, where many of the people who first migrated to Australia came from.

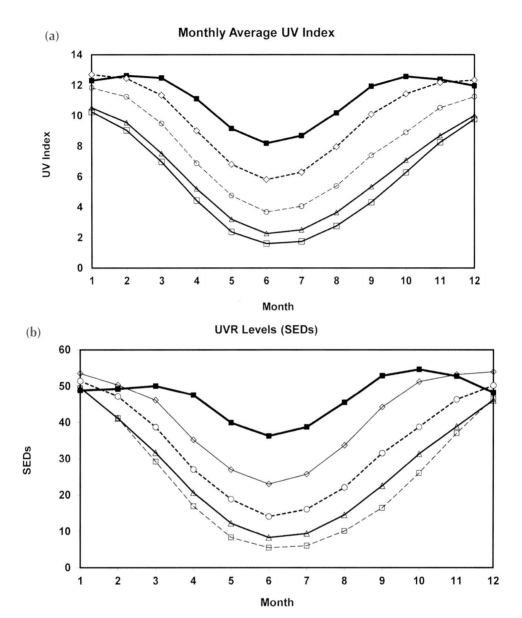

Fig. 2.9: (a) The monthly average peak UV Index in Darwin ■ (12°30'S), Townsville ◇ (19°10'S), Brisbane ○ (27°25'S), Sydney △ (33°55'S) and Melbourne □ (37°46'S). In summer the values are not dissimilar, but in winter the differences between Darwin and Townsville in the north and Sydney and Melbourne further south become substantial. Source: Measured by ARPANSA. (b) The monthly average total per day UVR in SEDs in Darwin ■ (12°30'S), Townsville ◇ (19°10'S), Brisbane ○ (27°25'S), Sydney △ (33°55'S) and Melbourne □ (37°46'S). Source: Measured by ARPANSA.

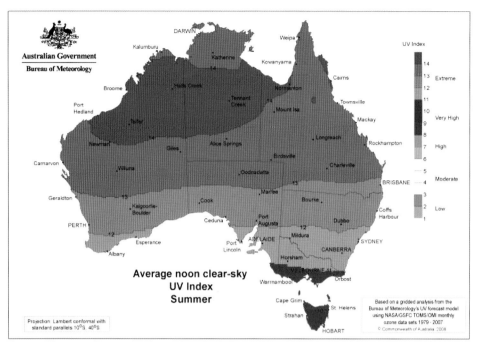

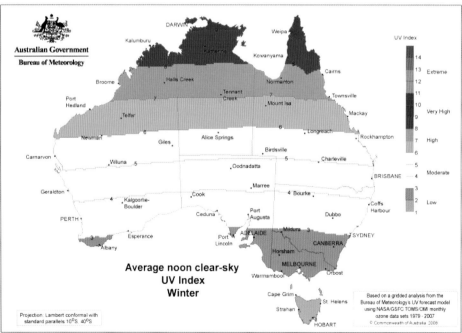

Fig. 2.10: Maps of Australia showing summer and winter average noon clear-sky UV Index levels. Locations in purple and red are the highest end of the UV Index level, and yellow and green are at the lowest. Permission granted by the Australian Bureau of Meteorology.

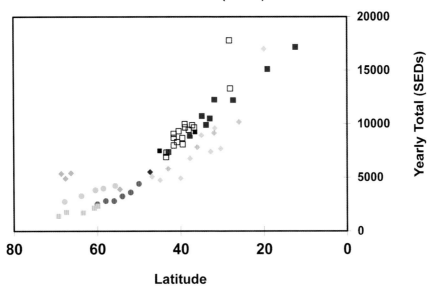

Fig. 2.11: The variation in annual solar UVR levels for several different countries: Australia ■, New Zealand ■, USA ◆, Spain □, Japan ◆, UK ●, Germany ◆, Sweden ●, Arctic sites ▥ and the Australian Antarctic stations ◆. The Spanish and US UV sites at low latitudes have higher levels of UVR than the Australian sites because they are at high altitude.

Those people would have been unprepared for the environment in Australia, particularly the levels of solar UVR. As a result, in the last 50 years Australia has had some of the highest incidences of skin cancer in the world. Many tourists from the Northern Hemisphere, who are inexperienced in dealing with high levels of solar UVR, are likely to use sun protective measures less than they need to and often end up with sunburn in Australia.

Another way to look at UV levels is to show a three-dimensional plot of measured solar UVR with the *x*-axis showing month of the year, the *y*-axis showing time of day and the colours showing the UV Index as defined by the colours used in the WHO UV Index publication.

These 3D plots show the maximum solar UVR levels for that location. Figure 2.12 shows some examples for different latitudes; the effect on the UV levels is obvious. The orange, red and purple colours signify very high and extreme levels of UVR. The more spread those colours, the longer those high levels of URV occur throughout the year in those locations.

It emphasises the SunSmart messages that began many years ago – Stay out of the sun between 10am and 3pm in summer! This is still true for each location for much of the year, but we can

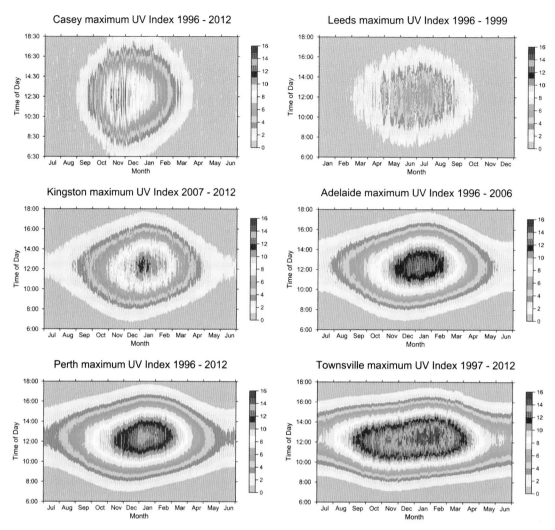

Fig. 2.12: 3D plots of the solar UV Index measurements at six locations with varying latitude. As the latitude decreases and the locations are closer to the equator, the length of time the UV Index is at higher levels increases dramatically, both during the day and during the year. For example, Kingston near Hobart has only a few months with UV Index levels above 10, while Townsville has UV Index levels above 10 for eight months. The UV Index levels of Leeds are included (courtesy of the National Radiological Protection Board, now Public Health England) to show the UV levels for a location in the Northern Hemisphere from which many people have emigrated to Australia.

also see that as we move closer to the equator, the hazards increase to higher levels and for longer time periods.

Artificial sources of UVR

Numerous artificial sources of UVR are used in many different applications in medical, industrial, scientific and domestic fields. Uses include sterilisation, photopolymerisation, photoactivation processes, psoriasis phototherapy and artificial suntanning. UVR is also present as a by-product in operations such as welding, glass processing, metal smelting and many processes involving incandescent materials. These sources generally emit a broad spectrum of wavelengths across the visible and much of the UVR spectrum. Some artificial sources of UVR with high UVB and UVC content such as arc welders can have threshold limit values (TLVs) of seconds (which means they are very intense source of UVR) to TLVs of more than 8 hours for standard (and much less intense) UVA sources, but this depends upon the exposure conditions as well as shielding and distance from the source. Most artificial sources of UVR used in the workplace are carefully controlled by a range of different methods.

Desk lighting (and domestic downlighting) involving the use of tungsten halogen lamps has been increasingly popular for several years. The lamps, containing a tungsten filament and a halogen gas (usually iodine), can emit significant levels of UVR. The halogen gas inside the bulb reduces evaporation of tungsten from the filament, which means the lamp will have a longer operational life.

These lamps are also operated at a higher temperature than ordinary lamps so the envelope must be quartz, which transmits UVR wavelengths, so the UV hazard must be controlled. The advantage is that a brighter light is produced from a lower power consumption, but the disadvantage is potentially hazardous levels of UVR emission.

These UVR levels are greater than allowed UVR exposure limits under certain exposure situations such as desk lighting, where people may be close to the lamps for extended periods of time. Tungsten halogen lamps generally now have an optical filter (e.g. 3 mm window glass) which substantially absorbs the UVR but transmits the visible radiation.

Fluorescent lamps

Until fairly recently, most lighting was either incandescent or low-pressure mercury lamps or fluorescent lamps, which use a fluorescent phosphor coating on the inside wall that converts mercury emission lines in the UVC at 189 nm and 254 nm to visible radiation that is useful for illumination. All lamps typically show the common mercury emission lines but the continuum emission depends upon the type of phosphor used. Hazardous UVB below 320 nm is generally blocked by the glass envelope. External diffusers attached to fluorescent lights also absorb UVR and further reduce UVR emissions.

Blacklights

Blacklights are fluorescent lights used in industry for the detection of flaws and cracks in materials. They predominately emit at 366 nm (in the UVA range) which causes fluorescence in various dyes lodged in the cracks of the material under examination. Occasionally the protective filter used to eliminate the visible light may crack and workers may be exposed to small amounts of unfiltered UVR, but as these emissions are in the UVA region the lamps are not generally a hazard. Low-power blacklights are also used for signature verification and in the entertainment industry, e.g. in nightclubs, to create unusual lighting effects. Their exposures are minimal and well below the recognised safe limits, therefore they are not a hazard to people using them or working all day in the vicinity.

Compact fluorescent lights

Compact fluorescent lights (CFLs) were introduced to replace energy-inefficient incandescent light globes (Fig. 2.13) but several people who were photosensitive (or had lupus) complained that they were experiencing side effects due to the small amount of UVR emitted by single-envelope CFLs. A large range of single-envelope and double-envelope CFLs available in Australia were

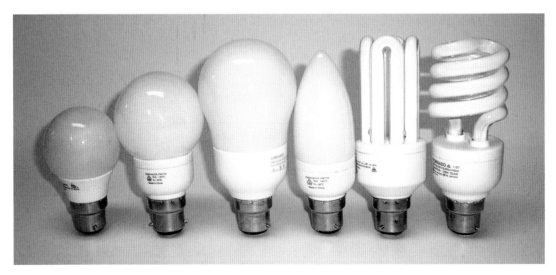

Fig. 2.13: Various types of CFLs. The four on the left are double envelopes, the two on the right are single envelopes (with the exposed fluoro tubes).

tested for emissions. While single-envelope CFLs emitted small amounts of UVR, the double envelopes emitted much less than incandescent globes. This is not an issue of concern for normal skin types, but it can be for people who are very photosensitive.

Welding

UVR emissions from arc welding are typically much greater than from the sun and are often extremely hazardous, both to the eyes because of the intensely bright arcs and to the skin from the UVR emissions. Some welders have been severely 'sunburned' because instead of wearing approved clothing designed to protect against welding they wore sun-protective clothing of UPF 50+. This was inadequate protection from the very intense UVR emissions from the welding operations. Research in the USA has demonstrated that, with new welding techniques, standard-issue clothing no longer provided sufficient protection against the increasingly intense welding sources. Specialised protective equipment is required for both the skin and the eyes when welding.

Light-emitting diodes

Light-emitting diodes (LEDs) are semiconductor devices that have similar features to other forms of lighting systems like tungsten halogen and fluorescent lights. They convert electrical current into light in a fairly efficient process that produces little heat compared to conventional lighting systems. It is possible to design LEDs to emit light in the UV, visible and near-infrared wavelengths. LED lamps or light globes are becoming common in home and industry for both general and special-purpose lighting.

There are solid-state UV LEDs which emit at specific wavelengths between 365 nm and 395 nm, generally referred to as blacklight LED's. More recently LEDs have been able to emit in the UVC wavelength region near 275–290 nm. These LEDs are used in purifying water and air and in curing polymers, but are difficult to manufacture. As UV LEDs are compact, use less power and are environmentally friendly and cost-effective they may eventually replace the traditional UV lamps in current use.

The main concern with UV LEDs is they commonly emit in a narrow angle (focused beam) and the UV damaging wavelengths cannot be seen until it is too late. Even looking into a high-intensity visible light LED may cause eye damage. At least with visible light LEDs the aversion response to intense light can come into play – a person will automatically look away due to discomfort. However, with UV LEDs the light emitted may be quite dim in the visible region, exposing people's eyes to UVR for potentially long periods. The symptoms of UVR exposure may not appear immediately, they may take several hours. When using UV LEDs appropriate UVR protective eyewear should be worn. When using lower-wavelength UV LEDs which can be hazardous (UVB or UVC), appropriate precautions need to be taken, e.g. shielding the source. UVR protective eyewear should be worn by anyone working in the vicinity.

Solaria

The use of solaria has been popular among some population groups wanting to tan (discussed in Chapter 3) but the scientific literature has shown a significant association between solarium use and skin cancer, both melanoma and non-melanoma. The 2002 Australian Standard on Solaria allowed an upper limit of intensity of UV Index 60 due to the demands of the solarium industry.

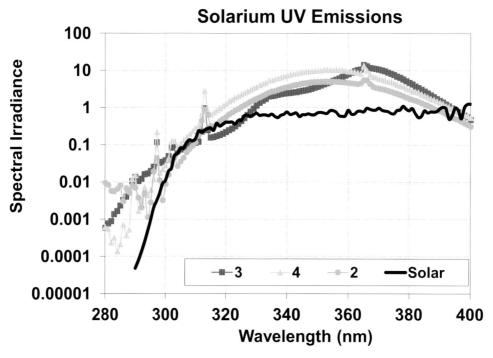

Fig. 2.14: Typical emissions of UVB and UVA from solaria in Australia. In the UVA region 330–380 nm the solarium emissions are a factor of 10 higher than those from the sun! In the UVB region below 300 nm the solarium emissions are also higher than those from the sun. Summer sunshine in Australia often has a UV Index of 12: solarium 2 had a UV Index of 20, solarium 3 had a UV Index of 30 and solarium 4 had a UV Index of 48 (in breach of the Solarium Standard AS/NZS 2635:2008, which set an upper limit of UV Index 36). From the end of 2014 commercial solaria services will be banned in Australia.

This meant that solaria were allowed to emit five times the intensity of normal summer sunlight in Australia (UV Index 12; Fig. 2.14). A survey showed that the emissions from solaria in Australia were among the highest in the world – added to the Australian population's already significant UVR exposure from the sun.

Incandescent sources

Incandescent sources (mostly used for lighting) were phased out a few years ago and are no longer imported into Australia, although people who are extremely photosensitive have stockpiled them for home use. These sources produce a continuous spectrum of optical radiation by heating a filament, usually tungsten, and are generally not very energy-efficient. However, their UVR emissions are low. The surface temperature of the filament determines the shape of the spectrum of radiation emitted: the higher the temperature the more UVR emitted, although the peak of the spectrum is invariably in the infrared.

Nail lamps

UV nail lamps are also a source of artificial UV radiation and are used to cure, harden and dry nail polish at home and in salons.

Studies have shown that UV nail lamps primarily emit UVA with no detectable UVB or UVC. The findings to date suggest that UV nail lamps do not significantly increase the lifetime risk of users developing basal cell or squamous cell carcinomas. The risk can be reduced to virtually zero by wearing fingerless gloves or applying sunscreen when the hands are being exposed.

Further reading

Gies P (2011) Ultraviolet radiation protection. In *Encyclopedia of Environmental Health*. (Ed. JO Nriagu) Vol. 5, pp. 483–495. Elsevier, Burlington.

Gies P, Roy C, Udelhofen P (2004) Solar and ultraviolet radiation. In *Prevention of Skin Cancer*. (Eds D Hill *et al.*) pp. 21–54. Kluwer Academic, Dordrecht.

Chapter 3

Tanning and solaria

Kimberley Dunstone, Jen Makin, Craig Sinclair and Suzanne Dobbinson

Key messages

- Tanned skin is a sign that the skin has been damaged by ultraviolet (UV) radiation.
- The desire for a tan is largely influenced by popular culture and has been in and out of fashion over time and in different cultures.
- There has been a decrease in the number of Australians seeking a tan in recent years.
- Solaria are devices that emit extreme doses of UV radiation and the World Health Organization recommends against using them as they increase cancer risk.
- Bans on commercial solaria come into force in Australia from the start of 2015.

What happens when skin tans?

Skin cells in the top layer of skin (epidermis) produce a pigment called melanin that gives skin its natural colour. When skin is exposed to UV radiation, more melanin is produced, causing the skin to darken. This is a 'tan'.

A tan is a sign that the skin is getting UV damage, even when no sunburn is experienced.

A tan offers very limited sunburn protection, usually similar to a sun protection factor (SPF) 3 sunscreen, depending on the skin type. However, a tan offers little, if any, protection against further DNA damage from UV radiation. For very fair-skinned people, no amount of sunbaking will protect from sunburn.

(a)

(b)

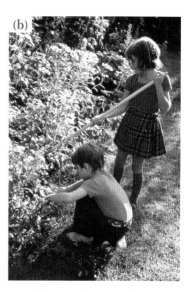
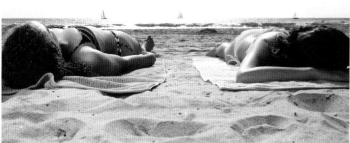

Fig. 3.1: (a) Tanning at the beach *v.* (b) working outside in the garden. (a) Reproduced with permission from Cancer Council Victoria. (b) Wellcome Library, London.

Many people do not deliberately sunbake but still get a tan through being out in the sun without sun protection during their daily activities, for example gardening or relaxing in the backyard, or walking along unshaded streets (Fig. 3.1). Whether the tan is deliberate or not, it is still a sign that the skin has been damaged.

Is the desire for a tan universal?

The desire to have a sun tan varies greatly between communities and cultures. For example, in many Asian countries pale skin continues to be popular, as reflected by the products available on pharmacy shelves. Instead of fake tanning lotions, artificial whitening creams are prominently displayed. There is research to show that attitudes to tanning change with changing cultural norms. For example, among first- and second-generation immigrants to the USA from Asia, tanning behaviours increase as they adopt the culture of their new home.

Tanned skin is a fashion that has also changed greatly over time. In Australia, the USA and Europe, pale skin was generally fashionable until the early 20th century, particularly among women of the upper social classes. Untanned skin was a sign that a person did not have to labour outside in the sun, so those who could afford to do so took care to avoid the sun and to protect themselves with clothing, hats, veils and parasols.

Deliberate sun tanning only really became popular from the late 1920s, as women began to engage in more outdoor leisure activities, attitudes to recreational swimming changed, clothing styles evolved to cover less skin, and scientific understanding of the positive effects of sunlight on diseases like tuberculosis grew (Fig. 3.2).

(a)

(b)

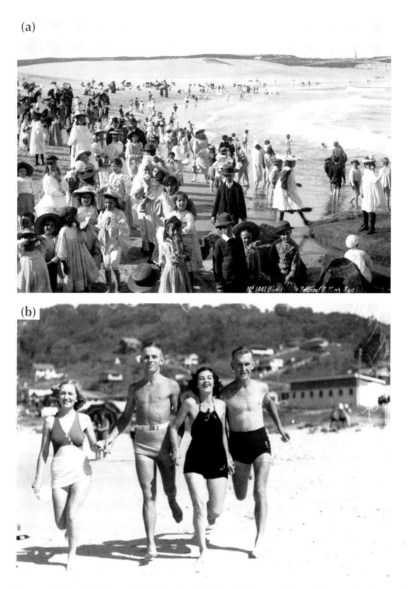

Fig. 3.2: Beachgoers (a) c.1900s and (b) in the 1930s. (a) Reproduced from the Powerhouse Museum Collection. Gift of Australian Consolidated Press under the Taxation Incentives for the Arts Scheme, 1985. (b) Reproduced from the State Library Queensland.

Understanding the risk of skin cancer due to excessive sun exposure also increased in the early 20th century, and physicians began to warn against the new trend of deliberate sunbathing. However, tanned skin has remained widely popular in western countries for several decades.

In Australia, there have been more recent changes in attitudes to tanning, following the introduction of public education campaigns to raise awareness of the link between UV radiation and skin cancer (Fig. 3.3). Since the 1980s, the percentage of people desiring a tan has decreased markedly, and dark tans in particular are much less popular.

However, skin cancer prevention campaigns to discourage tanning must still compete with widespread portrayal of tans as attractive in magazines, films and television programming. Australian research has shown, for example, that models in popular women's magazines often contradict public health messages concerning skin cancer prevention, as they are rarely shown

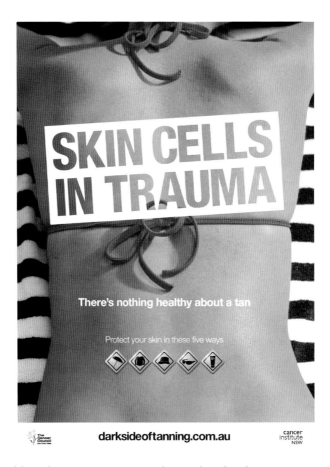

Fig. 3.3: A recent public education campaign, The Dark Side of Tanning. Reproduced with permission from Cancer Institute NSW.

wearing hats or in the shade. The proportion of models portrayed with moderate to dark tans decreased from the late 1980s, but then increased again. The research suggests that exposure to images of tanned models may both promote and reflect real women's tanning beliefs and behaviour.

What are the trends in desirability of tanning?

Encouragingly, evidence from state and national surveys (Table 3.1) of Australian's sun-related attitudes and behaviours conducted across many years shows a shift in people's attitudes and behaviours over the decades.

In Victoria these surveys have been conducted since 1987, when the majority of Victorians surveyed preferred a suntan. In 1990 soon after the launch of SunSmart Victorians' preference for a tan rapidly decreased, but there was a weakening of this improvement in population attitudes during 1997–2001. These changes were correlated with the amount of exposure to SunSmart TV advertising.

On a national scale these surveys have been conducted since 2003, and the trend is similar. The percentage of people who like to get a suntan decreased during the time of the national media campaign across seven years among both Australian adolescents (from 60% in 2003 to 45% in

Table 3.1: Trends in adolescents' and adults' intentional tanning attitudes and behaviour

Outcome	Adolescents (*N* = 2718)			Adults (*N* = 15 570)		
	2003–04 % *N* = 699	2006–07 % *N* = 652	2010–11 % *N* = 1367	2003–04 % *N* = 5073	2006–07 % *N* = 5085	2010–11 % *N* = 5412
Prefer a suntan	60	51	45	39	32	27
Believe suntanned person *looks* more healthy	41	43	36	50	46	42
Believe suntanned person *is* more healthy	19	17	12	14	12	10
Perceive friends think a suntan is a good thing	77	71	66	42	37	36
Attempted a suntan this season	32	22	22	15	11	9

Source: Volkov *et al.* (2013).

2011) and adults (from 39% in 2003 to 27% in 2011). There has been a corresponding decrease in the percentage of people who deliberately attempted a suntan among both Australian adolescents (from 32% in 2003 to 22% in 2011) and adults (from 15% in 2003 to 9% in 2011).

Is it okay to get a tan if you don't deliberately sunbake?

It is not only people who deliberately sunbake or use a solarium who get a tan – many people also get a tan through their normal, daily, incidental exposure. Everyday exposure if no sun protection is used, whether at an outside café, a BBQ, gardening at home or just spending time at the park, all adds up and increases the risk of skin damage.

Most Australians have got the message that deliberate tanning is dangerous, however many also think it's okay if they get unintentionally tanned while just going about their everyday activities. This is not true. Whether getting a tan is deliberate or not, tanned skin is a sign of skin damage and overexposure to UV radiation.

'Tanorexia', or tanning addiction

Studies of frequent tanners have suggested possible links between tanning behaviour and dependence and addiction. Studies suggest that UV radiation is a reinforcing stimulus, as frequent tanners can distinguish when exposed to UV and non-UV under blinded conditions. When given the option they choose to undertake further UV exposure. There is evidence that frequent tanners show signs of addiction similar to those used as criteria for substance abuse or dependence, including developing withdrawal symptoms and having difficulty controlling their use. Frequent tanning may also produce a release of endorphins when the skin is exposed to UV radiation. As endorphins are a type of natural opioid involved in the brain's reward pathway, their release creates a future incentive to tan.

Increased sun sensitivity in people taking some medication or wearing cosmetics

Some cosmetics and prescription medications can increase the sensitivity of the skin to UV radiation. These include anti-depressants, antibiotics, drugs for high blood pressure, some medicines for skin conditions, drugs that suppress the immune system and some anti-inflammatory drugs and creams.

Exposure to UV radiation after taking these drugs or using cosmetics may decrease the time it takes for the skin to burn and may cause an allergic skin reaction. This can be serious and in some cases life-threatening, requiring hospitalisation.

Tan accelerators

Tan accelerators are available in tablet or lotion form and claim to stimulate the production of melanin (the pigment that is responsible for skin colour) in the body. These accelerators often contain the chemicals psoralen and tyrosine. Psoralen should be used only under medical supervision to treat skin problems such as psoriasis.

When melanin cells are sensitised it may be possible to get a suntan in a shorter time than usual; however, the increased sensitivity may also cause severe sunburn. There is a lack of scientific data showing that tanning accelerators are effective. There is also little information on the safety of use of many such products.

Spray-on tans: a safe alternative?

Fake tans are available as creams or lotions for use at home, or as spray tans from salons or mobile services. Fake tans simulate a suntan by dyeing the outer layer of skin. It is important to remember that fake tans do not provide sun protection – even though some may contain a limited SPF, this will only be effective for the first couple of hours after applying the product, just like a sunscreen. All tanning products should be used in conjunction with the five sun protection measures – clothing, sunscreen, wide-brimmed hat, shade and sunglasses.

Some concern has been raised about the safety of spray tans and more studies on their safety are required. Researchers in the USA have expressed concerns over the potential inhalation of substances such as dihydroxyacetone (DHA) during a spray tan, as a result of tests carried out on cells in the laboratory. It has been suggested that the potential risk can be reduced by using goggles and a mask to protect against inhaling during a spray tan, or by using topical creams or lotions which cannot be inhaled. If any such risk does exist, it is also a concern for those working in salons where the spray tans are applied as they are likely to have repeated exposure.

Myths about tanning

Tanning is a sign I'm getting my vitamin D. NOT TRUE

Tanning is a sign that your skin is being damaged. Most Australians receive enough vitamin D while doing normal day-to-day activities. When you are exposed to UV radiation, you only make vitamin D for a short amount of time – staying exposed for longer periods of time doesn't increase vitamin D levels further (see Chapter 8).

Solaria should never be used to boost vitamin D levels as they emit dangerous levels of UV which increase the risk of skin cancer.

Although UV radiation does stimulate synthesis of vitamin D, only the UVB component of UV radiation is responsible for vitamin D synthesis. Exposing your skin to extreme levels of UV radiation through a solarium is not safe and solaria mostly emit UVA which has no effect on skin vitamin D synthesis.

If I build up my tan, I'll be protected from the sun. NOT TRUE

It is a myth that getting a tan will protect your skin from burning in the sun. Laboratory tests on people have shown a tan to be equivalent to a sunscreen with an SPF of 3 – it therefore offers only minimal protection.

A tan won't protect skin from further damage when you're out in the sun and exposed to UV radiation. Tans offer no protection against genetic damage to skin cells, which can occur without burning. A tan increases your risk of skin cancer and premature ageing.

Research has also shown that a tan does not reduce the chance of getting sunburnt when spending time outdoors. It appears that a false sense of protection from a 'base tan' encourages people to increase their time in the sun.

A tan is healthy. NOT TRUE

A tan is a sign that the skin is getting UV radiation damage. It is not a sign of good health.

Some may argue that a tan gives a healthy-looking glow. The skin pigment darkening that follows exposure to UV radiation may indeed hide existing imperfections such as small wrinkles and other blemishes, but the effect will not last for long. The skin imperfections will be obvious again and in fact be accelerated by exposure to intense UV radiation.

My skin is damaged only if I get burnt. NOT TRUE

Tanning without burning can still cause skin damage and premature skin ageing and can increase the risk of skin cancer. UV radiation can cause irreparable DNA damage. Each time skin is exposed to UV radiation from the sun or from a solarium, the risk of developing skin cancer is increased.

What are solaria?

A solarium is a tanning unit that a person might use to tan their skin using artificial UV radiation (Fig. 3.4). Other names for solaria are sunbeds, sunlamps, indoor or artificial tanning beds and tanning booths.

Solaria (the plural of solarium) use an array of fluorescent lamps to focus UV radiation on a person lying under a canopy or clam-shaped structure. A tanning booth is similar except that the person stands while tanning. Exposure to UV radiation causes darkening of the melanin to produce a tan. People who sunburn and can't get a tan in the sun will also not tan in a solarium.

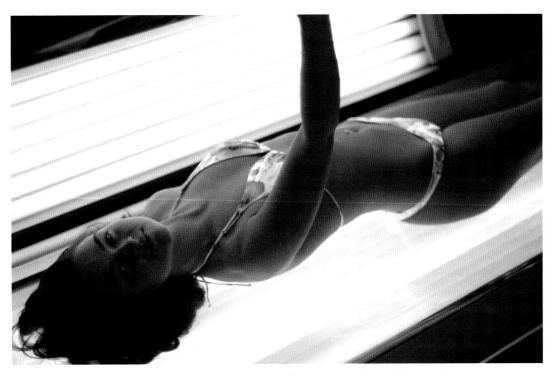

Fig. 3.4: A solarium. Reproduced with permission from Cancer Council Australia.

Why do solaria pose a health risk?

Overexposure to UV radiation from the sun and artificial sources, such as solaria, plays an important role in the development of several skin and eye conditions. These include premature skin ageing, skin cancer, cataracts and other eye conditions. Overexposure to UV radiation is also linked to suppression of the immune system. The damage associated with solarium use has been well documented in international and national studies; solarium use has been linked to an increased risk of all three main types of skin cancer.

The bottom line is that no solarium can provide a safe tan. The UV radiation given out by a solarium is a different type and intensity from that generated by the sun. Solaria emit both UVA and UVB radiation but the ratio between them differs from that of the sun. So does the intensity – solaria emissions are many times stronger than those from the midday summer sun.

The greater UV intensity, along with a high proportion of skin exposed, means that during a typical solarium session users are exposed to a dose of UV radiation well above anything they would have experienced in the outdoors (see Chapter 2, p. 48).

In 2009, the International Agency for Research on Cancer moved UV-emitting tanning beds to its highest cancer risk category, labelling them as carcinogenic to humans. In line with this, the World Health Organization does not recommend the use of artificial tanning for cosmetic rather than medical use.

Regulation of solaria

From 2008, the solarium industry in Australia was regulated on a state-by-state basis, i.e. to ban the use of solaria by people under 18 and adults with highly sensitive skin (that burns easily and does not tan). Given the growing scientific evidence of the strong link between sunbed use and skin cancer risk, since 2012 all Australian states and territories have declared or foreshadowed an outright ban on solaria to be introduced at the start of 2015.

Australia is only the second country in the world to announce outright bans on solaria for cosmetic purposes, after Brazil introduced a ban in 2009. The bans result from a combination of years of research and the active advocacy of prominent academics, cancer organisations and grassroots community campaigners. The personal stories of two individuals were particularly influential in changing public opinion and convincing governments first to legislate, and then to ban solaria.

Clare Oliver was a young woman in Melbourne who attributed her melanoma to solarium use in her early 20s. She died at 26, after her active campaign against solaria attracted a great deal of media attention. The Victorian government announced legislation soon after her death, followed by the other states and territories, which banned solarium access for people under 18 years old and people with pale skin.

Jay Allen's campaign to ban solariums in NSW and around the country began when he was diagnosed with melanoma in 2007. The young father of two used social and traditional media, a community petition and directly lobbied politicians to call for a ban. He was supported by Cancer Council NSW, the NSW Greens political party and a prominent public health academic, Professor Simon Chapman.

As long as solaria are available to the public, there is a need for guidelines or legislation to reduce the risks associated with their use. By reducing solarium use, future cases of skin cancer can be prevented, along with the associated disease, health care costs and, in some cases, death.

There are fears that as solaria are prohibited in several states and territories in Australia, there may be a rise in commercial solaria for sale and possible purchase by the general public. In some states, buyback schemes and safe disposal processes are being put in place to ensure the tanning machines are taken out of circulation. Using a solarium at home without supervision can be hazardous, as a person may use it excessively. In addition, if there is no monitoring or maintenance (which is unlikely in the home situation), there is no way to know or control the amount of UV radiation emitted by a tanning machine.

Further reading

Boniol M, Autier P, Boyle P, Gandini S (2012) Cutaneous melanoma attributable to sunbed use: systematic review and meta-analysis. *British Medical Journal (Clinical Research Edn)* **345**, e4757 [published erratum appears in BMJ 2012,345]. Abstract available at http://www.ncbi. nlm.nih.gov/pubmed/22833605

Cancer Council Victoria (2013) Solariums Position Statement. Last updated 27 June 2013. Accessed 29 July 2013. http://wiki.cancer.org.au/prevention/Position_statement_-_Solariums.

Cust AE, Armstrong BK, Goumas C, Jenkins MA, Schmid H, Hopper JL, *et al.* (2011) Sunbed use during adolescence and early adulthood is associated with increased risk of early-onset melanoma. *International Journal of Cancer* **128**(10), 2425–2435. Abstract available at http:// www.ncbi.nlm.nih.gov/pubmed/2066923210.1002/ijc.25576

International Agency for Research on Cancer Working Group on artificial ultraviolet (UV) light and skin cancer(2007) The association of use of sunbeds with cutaneous malignant melanoma and other skin cancers: a systematic review. *International Journal of Cancer* **120**(5), 1116–1122. Abstract available at http://www.ncbi.nlm.nih.gov/pubmed/17131335

Joint Standards Australia/Standards New Zealand Committee CS-064 (2008) *AS/NZS 2635:2008. Solaria for Cosmetic Purposes.* Standards Australia/Standards New Zealand, Sydney/Wellington.

Volkov A, Dobbinson S, Wakefield M, Slevin T (2013) Seven-year trends in sun protection and sunburn among Australian adolescents and adults. *Australia and New Zealand Journal of Public Health* **37**(1), 63–69.

Chapter 4

UV protection by clothing, hats and umbrellas

Peter Gies, Alan McLennan and John Javorniczky

Key messages

- Hats, clothing and shade can afford people good levels of protection from ultraviolet radiation (UVR) exposure, especially when the protective equipment meets the Australian Standards and guidelines for UVR protection.
- Clothing should have good body coverage, e.g. collars, ¾ sleeves and longer shorts. Darker colours give better sun protection, as do closely woven fabrics. Sun protection values in some fabrics may diminish with repeated washing (40 washes is approximately the lifetime for many garments) and wet fabric often gives reduced sun protection.
- Hats with a broad brim (7.5 cm or larger) or legionnaire's hats provide the best sun protection. As with clothing, good fabric selection is important.
- Personal, beach or market umbrellas can be helpful to add shade but diffuse and reflected UVR exposure can diminish the effect of umbrella shade.
- Man-made shade is an increasingly popular form of sun protection. Again, selecting the right fabric is vital to ensure effective protection. Most shadecloth is designed for horticultural use and does not provide good UV protection for humans.

In summer in Australia on a sunny day, a fair-skinned person outside and unprotected around the middle of the day could receive enough solar UVR in 10–15 minutes to cause sunburn. If you do make the effort of protecting yourself and your family from the sun, it is a good idea to make sure the products you use will do the job well.

Fabrics differ enormously in their ability to cut down UVR. A big sombrero with a 30 cm wide brim might seem great, but if the weave of the straw has strands as far apart as chicken coop wire, lots of UVR will still penetrate. Similarly, a woollen swimsuit might sound like great sun protection, but if it takes the form of a crochet bikini, you can expect some serious sunburn on unprotected skin.

Here we look at what works well, and what is not so good in protecting human skin from the ravages of the sun.

What type of clothing is best?

As far as sun protection goes, the best clothing has two important features:

- it covers a lot of a person's skin;
- it strongly reduces the amount of UVR getting through to their skin.

A long-sleeved shirt will provide much more coverage than a T-shirt and long pants will cover more exposed skin than shorts. We all know that skin that has been covered for much of a person's lifetime shows much less sun damage and skin ageing than areas of skin that are almost always exposed. Clothing is one of the important five elements of sun protection: the others are hats, shade, sunglasses and sunscreens, which are discussed in other chapters of this book.

Hats, particularly those with a wide brim, will help protect more of the face and ears than the ever-popular baseball cap. Sunglasses, particularly in Australia, can help protect the eyes and the areas around the eyes. We can be more confident here as Australia has the world's only mandatory sunglass standard (see Chapter 7) that all sunglasses sold in Australia must comply with. Shade is becoming much more available in public places and sunscreen is really useful for covering the areas of skin that can be otherwise hard to protect, such as the face and hands.

What makes a difference: the role of fabric weave

If you are going to protect yourself by wearing clothing that covers much of your skin, then you should also consider how protective the clothing is for your skin. That is, the clothing fabric or material needs to strongly block UVR from the sun.

If you look closely at a fabric you can often see that there are spaces between the fibres where light (and UVR) can get through. The tighter and closer together the fibres, the less the rays of sunlight can pass through. Fabrics with large spaces between the fibres and with open weaves provide much less protection against solar UVR than tightly woven fabrics.

Clothing can be made from many different fibres, such as cotton, nylon, polyester or wool, and these fibres will absorb some or perhaps all of the UVR. Figure 4.1 shows the weaves of four fabrics with different weave densities and different measured ultraviolet protection factors (UPFs) ranging from UPF4 for the most open weave up to UPF50 for the most tightly woven. The UPF is explained below.

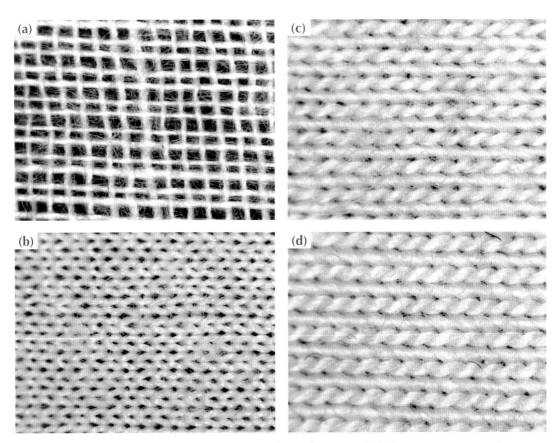

Fig. 4.1: Examples of the weave and structure of four fabrics with different UPF ratings, showing the effect the tightness of the weave or knit has on the measured UPFs. Sample A is woven and has a UPF of 4, Sample B has a UPF of 10, Sample C has a UPF of 25 and Sample D has a UPF of 50. Samples B, C and D are all knitted.

In the clothing industry, the term 'cover factor' denotes how much of the fabric surface area contains fibres. Different fabrics may have identical cover factors but one fabric may have denser fibres which will affect the weight of the fabric. The more of the fabric surface that is solid material, the less open space there is for the sun's rays to pass through.

The construction of the fabric is the way the fibres are linked together within the fabric and that can affect how close together the fibres can be. Most clothing is either of knitted or woven construction. The construction plays an important role as it determines whether the amount of open space in a garment changes when tension is applied or when the fabric is washed. Knitted fabrics usually stretch more than woven fabrics.

What the fibres are made of also affects the measured UV protection, as some fibres completely block UVR and others can transmit or reflect some of the UVR. Synthetic fibres such as rayon, nylon, polyester or acrylic, can strongly absorb UVR. The weight of the material as well as its weave density can also play a big role in how much UVR is blocked. Dense fabrics such as denim will block more UVR than thin lightweight fabrics.

What is SPF/UPF and why do I need to know?

Most people have heard of the SPF (sun protection factor) as it applies to sunscreen. In Chapter 5 we focus on sunscreens and the meaning of SPF is explained there. In simple terms, SPF is a measure of the increase in the amount of time sunscreen allows you to be in the sun before your skin burns. If your unprotected skin takes 10 minutes to burn in the summer sun, effectively applied sunscreen of SPF30 will mean you will have 30×10 minutes before burning occurs.

The UPF is a similar concept. If fabric is rated UPF50, as many fabrics are, skin covered by that fabric will take 50×10 minutes (500 minutes) before burning occurs.

Ultraviolet protection factor or UPF was chosen to differentiate it from SPF when the first Sun Protective Clothing Standard was introduced in Australia in 1996. The UPF test uses a scientifically determined response of human skin to solar UVR and calculates the effectiveness of fabrics against a solar UVR spectrum.

Most of the testing for UPF for clothing, hats and many other products conducted in Australia is done by the Australian Radiation Protection and Nuclear Safety Agency (ARPANSA), an Australian government agency based in Melbourne. Most of the measurements reported in this chapter were made by ARPANSA.

Ageing, stretching fabric and sun protection

In Australia, UPF tests are generally carried out on fabrics that are in new condition as required by the current clothing standard. After their first wash many cotton-based fabrics shrink slightly, which makes the gaps between the fibres smaller and therefore more difficult for UVR to be transmitted. This generally remains the case for the first 40 washes but further washing may affect some fabrics, fading colours and reducing the fibres so that the UPF rating will become lower.

Additives to improve sun protection: a way to go?

It is possible to add chemical compounds such as optical whitening agents and UV-cutting compounds to fabrics, which will increase their UVR protection. These compounds are sometimes added during production at the fabric mill by treating the fabric. They can also be added later as domestic wash-in additives. UV-cutting agents can absorb strongly in the lower parts of the spectrum (e.g. the highly sunburning UVB area) and can substantially increase a fabric's UVR protection under the right conditions. The success of the uptake of the UV-cutting agents depends on both the type of agents as well as the material they are applied to. Washing powders with optical brighteners have been demonstrated to increase the UV protection of clothing.

Does colour make a difference?

In general, darker colours absorb UVR more strongly than lighter colours. In years of testing the UVR protection of fabrics at ARPANSA, there have been many occasions when the same base fabric was submitted for testing in a range of different colours. As a general rule, the darker colours absorbed more strongly than the lighter colours so they had higher measured protection against UVR. For example, in one set of materials made from the same base fabric, the black rated as 250 (i.e. UPF50+), the blue rated at 80 (UPF50+) and the red rated at 150 (UPF50+) while the lighter colours such as white rated at UPF22, oatmeal rated at UPF16 and pale blue rated at UPF13. The effect of colour is valid for cotton fabrics as well as polyester fabrics of the same weave and weight.

The design is the thing: how much skin is covered

Your skin will only be protected against the sun if it is covered. Body coverage is something that is being considered in the revised Australian Sun Protective Clothing Standard, with the idea that claims of sun protection can only be made for garments that actually cover sufficient areas of the body. The question is, what is sufficient? Obviously, shirts with collars help protect the neck area and long sleeves give better protection than short or no sleeves.

Getting wet: clothing in the water – rashies, bathers, cossies, bikinis and budgie smugglers

When a garment is wet its UVR protection may be lower. The amount the UPF rating drops when a garment is wet depends upon the type of fabric and the amount of moisture it absorbs. Tests showed that the average measured UPF for a set of white T-shirts reduced to 50% of the UPF when the shirts were wet. The effect is much less with elastane or lycra garments designed to be used in the surf or on the beach where there was only a slight reduction in measured UPF for some samples and most showed little or no reduction in measured UPF. 'Rashies' were originally promoted as a way of reducing friction rash to the chest and stomach while body-boarding. Now they are commonly used as very effective sun protection garments when swimming or around water.

Hats and skin cancer

Is a hat really just a hat? The broad-brimmed hat *v.* the bucket hat and the baseball cap

Hats can provide extra protection to the head and face but the design of the hat is important. Hats can be a useful addition to the application of sunscreen to the face and head, but will rarely provide sufficient protection on their own to anyone outside in summer when solar UVR levels are high. This is because, although they provide protection to different areas of the head, neck and face, the protection factors (PFs) due to the shading effect of the hat are rarely double figures (e.g. 10–15). More often they are only single figures, e.g. 2–4. To provide good sun protection PFs of at least 15 are required.

Several studies have looked at the amount of protection provided to different areas of the face such as the nose, forehead, cheeks, neck and ears and found that it can vary significantly depending upon the type of hat and the design, e.g. how broad is the brim? Broad-brimmed hats (e.g. hats for adults with a brim of 7.5 cm or more) perform better at shading more of the facial areas than baseball caps. Caps provide reasonable protection to the scalp, forehead and nose but almost none to any of the other sites such as the ears. Table 4.1 shows the amount of protection provided to different areas of the head by four types of hats (see also Fig. 4.2).

Table 4.1: PFs for various facial and head sites from four types of hats

Hat type	Forehead	Cheeks	Nose	Ears	Chin	Neck
Brimmed	15+	2–3	6–8	6–8	>1	~2
Bucket	15	2–3	6–7	6–8	>1	~2
Baseball cap	8–10	>1	4–5	>1	>1	>1
Legionnaire's cap	13	1–6	10	4–5	>1	>4

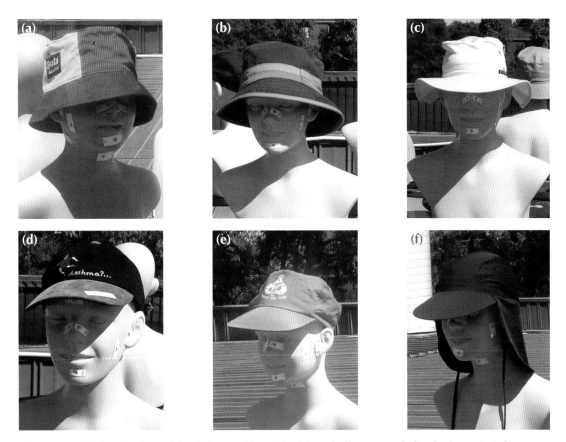

Fig. 4.2: (a, b) Bucket hats, (c) a brimmed hat, (d, e) baseball caps and (f) a legionnaire's hat being tested for their UV protection using UV-sensitive film patches. The figures clearly show that while the baseball caps shade and protect the nose and forehead, they provide little protection to the ears and cheeks. The bucket hats and brimmed hat as well as the legionnaire's hat provide shading and protection to more of the face and neck.

Different levels of sun protection from different kinds of hats

As we have made clear, in summer in Australia on a sunny day a fair-skinned person outside and unprotected would receive enough solar UVR in 10–15 minutes to cause sunburn. If they wore a hat with a PF of 2 or 3, they would need to be outside for two to three times as long (i.e. 20–45 minutes) to get sunburned. Expressed another way, if they were outside for 10–15 minutes with a hat with PFs of 2 or 3, they would get a UVR dose two or three times smaller. So, although hats are helpful, sunscreen will be required if that person is outside for more than 10–20 minutes.

While hats are mostly useful against the direct sun, when it is cloudy there is more indirect and scattered solar UVR. The protection provided by hats can be lessened in such conditions.

Does hat fabric matter?

What the hat is made of can be important – the hat material must block solar UVR. Most of the materials used in hats provide excellent protection against UVR as they naturally block or absorb it. Straw hats can have spaces between the individual fibres, but they also provide comfort and fashion and allow air circulation. Often a second inner layer of material is used to provide extra protection and comfort. If buying a straw hat, look for one with a fabric lining.

Choosing a hat

In many cases hats are a personal statement – different people like to wear different types of hats. When choosing a hat we should consider the amount of sun protection it offers, whether it is practical, fashion trends, costs, safety and ventilation. In Chapter 13 we look at who does or does not wear hats in Australia, what kinds and why.

Umbrellas

Umbrellas, both the personal types and larger ones such as beach umbrellas, can be useful in providing extra protection against the sun. First, it is important that the material the umbrellas are made of blocks UVR, so the shading they provide from the direct sun is free from UVR. However, unless the umbrellas are of a substantial size the amount of protection will be minimal as they are particularly poor at protecting against diffuse UVR from the sky (see Chapters 2 and 6 regarding direct and diffuse UVR).

Spanish researchers looked at the amount of protection provided by a beach umbrella and found that it intercepted all direct UV irradiance, but only part of the diffuse component. They found that the PF of the umbrella against solar UVR was only 3 and even that depended upon how close to the canopy the person was. The greater the distance between the person and the canopy, the greater the amount of UVR exposure.

Shadecloth

Chapter 6 examines the issue of shade in detail. The fabric used when providing man-made shade is important. Various types of fabrics and shadecloth material can be used for shade structures. Fabrics such as canvas, sailcloth and awning or umbrella fabric are generally tightly woven and can block up to 99% of UVR.

The Australian Standard for synthetic shadecloth (AS 4174 – 1994) is designed for agricultural and horticultural industries and is aimed at providing optimum growing conditions for a variety of plants. However, shadecloth is also widely used in Australia in other applications, in particular to provide a barrier to solar UVR for people enjoying outdoor activities.

Shadecloths designed for horticultural purposes generally have PFs less than 10, but some are available with PF ratings of 50 and higher.

In recent years there has been an increase in the use of shadecloth by kindergartens, schools and councils to provide comfortable outdoor shaded areas during the day. The shadecloth standard is currently under revision and the scope of the updated standard will address the use of shadecloth materials in shade structures, which are now an essential part of any sun protection strategy.

What about glass?

Most glass can provide good levels of UVR protection. The amount of protection is influenced by the thickness of the glass, the type and colour of the glass. UVB radiation is almost completely blocked by most types of glass. Laminated glass also blocks almost all UVA while annealed and tempered glass blocks 70–75% of UVA.

Glass in cars

Laminated glass such as that used in car windscreens provides high PFs of over 50. Side windows provide less UV protection – often at levels of about PF12–14. Tinting vehicle side windows can increase the PF to more than 50. It is possible to have a clear film (and some dark tints) applied that will virtually eliminate all solar UVR including the UVA.

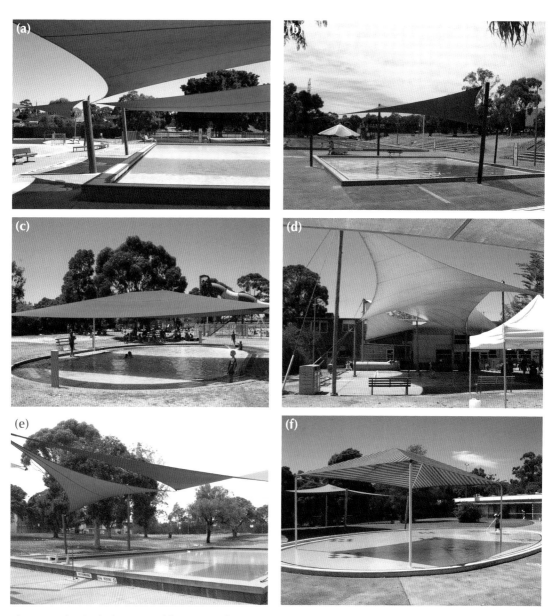

Fig. 4.3: Shadecloth material being used over public swimming pools in Melbourne to provide shade and protection from the sun.

Conclusion

The major advantage of fabric-based sun protection, clothing, hats, umbrellas, shadecloth and glass is that there is a physical barrier between UVR and the skin. Another advantage is it is easy to see where the protection covers, and where it does not. However, as shown here, a range of factors influence the level of protection. Nonetheless, these are some of the best ways to protect our skin from the harsh Australian sun.

Further reading

Gies P (2007) Photoprotection by clothing. *Photodermatology, Photoimmunology and Photomedicine* **23**, 264–274. doi:10.1111/j.1600-0781.2007.00309.x.

The Shade Handbook. Your local state Cancer Council.

Chapter 5

'Slop on some sunscreen': the mysteries and truth about sunscreen

Brian Diffey

Key messages

- Regular sunscreen use has been proven to reduce the chance of getting common or non-melanoma skin cancers and there is some evidence of reducing melanoma risk, but more evidence is needed.
- Modern sunscreen formulations are improving both their cosmetic feel and their capacity to protect the skin.
- Sunscreen is not a suit of armour against the sun. It is rarely applied in sufficient quantity or frequency to achieve the sun protection on the label. It can rub or wash off or sections of skin can be missed.
- Sunscreen is useful but it should not be considered the only or the major strategy for skin cancer prevention.

What is a sunscreen?

A sunscreen is a substance applied to the skin to reduce the intensity of the sun's ultraviolet (UV) rays entering the skin and damaging skin cells. Sunscreens can take many forms including creams, milks, lotions, gels, foams, oils, ointments and sprays. The active ingredients of a sunscreen are normally one to six (occasionally more) chemicals that can either absorb UV radiation and convert it into harmless warmth (so weak that we can't feel it), or scatter the UV rays away from the skin and so prevent them entering the skin and causing harm.

In addition to these active chemicals, several other chemicals called excipients are used to give the product its particular cosmetic feel. Some sunscreens may contain additional chemicals such as antioxidants that can play some role in reducing UV damage to the skin.

When were sunscreens first used?

The first use of sunscreens was reported in 1928 in the USA, and in the early 1930s a product containing phenyl salicylate as the active ingredient appeared on the Australian market. Sunscreens were first used not so much to protect the skin from harm as to encourage tanning by reducing the risk of burning, as the advertisement from the 1930s shows (Fig. 5.1).

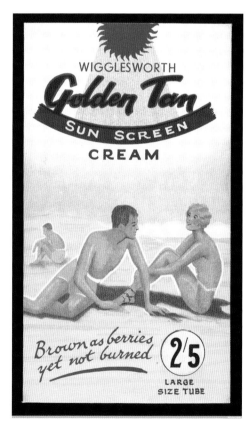

Fig. 5.1: A 1930s advertisement for a sunscreen. Wellcome Library, London.

Since those early days, sunscreens have become increasingly popular, particularly during outdoor recreation in which as little clothing is worn as possible, such as at the beach. Sunscreens are widely available and are mostly distributed in supermarkets and in pharmacies as over-the-counter products. They are also sold directly by doctors (e.g. in the USA), by hospitals (e.g. in Italy) and by cancer control organisations and cancer charities like the Cancer Council. In Australia, sunscreens are commonly available in the workplace as part of occupational health and safety programs, and are widely available in schools since their use by children is actively promoted. In contrast, in the USA, partly because of fear of litigation, schools rarely promote sunscreens as they are classified as drugs.

Who uses sunscreens?

Surveys generally find that sunscreens are more likely to be used by women than by men, by higher socio-economic groups, and by younger and middle-aged people rather than elderly people. People are more likely to have bought or used a sunscreen if there are children in their home, and if their skin is white rather than brown or black.

Why do people use (and not use) sunscreens?

By far the most common reason that people give for using sunscreen is to protect against sunburn. Other reasons include:

- knowing the dangers of sun exposure;
- perceiving themselves as at high risk of skin cancer;
- knowing people who had skin cancer;
- protecting against ageing and wrinkling;
- extending time in the sun;
- previously had skin cancer.

We should not forget that many people do not use sunscreens regularly or at all. The reasons that people give for choosing not to apply sunscreens to their skin include:

- having skin that does not burn easily;
- already have a 'protective' tan;
- takes too much time to apply;
- not outdoors enough to warrant use;

- nuisance and greasy to apply;
- feels hot and sweaty;
- expensive;
- retards desired tan;
- use other sun protective measures;
- forgetting.

The sun protection factor

The concept of the sun protection factor (SPF) was popularised by Austrian scientist Franz Greiter in the 1970s and subsequently adopted by many regulatory authorities and the cosmetic and pharmaceutical industries. It is commonly interpreted as 'how much longer skin covered with sunscreen takes to burn compared with unprotected skin'. So if you burn after 10 minutes in the sun, then using a sunscreen labelled with, e.g. SPF30, is taken to mean that you can safely remain in the sun for $10 \times 30 = 300$ minutes (= five hours) before burning.

This definition focuses on extending time in the sun. A better way of thinking about the SPF is that if you spend a certain time in the sun, then wearing a sunscreen with a given SPF reduces the UV dose to 1/SPF of that you would have received by spending the same time in the sun with no sunscreen applied. So applying an SPF30 sunscreen results in a UV exposure to the skin 1/30th of that you would have received if you had not applied any sunscreen. However, this statement is true *only* if the sunscreen is providing protection equivalent to the SPF. As we shall see later, this rarely happens – most people who apply sunscreen are protected to a much lesser extent than they realise.

Twenty-five years ago most commercially available sunscreen products had SPFs less than 10 but by 2000 most manufacturers produced products with factors of 15–30. It is not uncommon to find products today claiming an SPF of 50 or higher. In Australia, as of late 2012, the maximum SPF claim permitted was 50 plus (50+).

Active ingredients

The heart of any sunscreen product is the ingredient that protects you from the sun's UV rays. It is known as the 'active ingredient(s)' and is commonly referred to as the UV absorber or UV filter. UV filters may be classified as inorganic chemicals or organic chemicals.

Inorganic UV filters

These are chemicals that scatter UV radiation away from the skin. Examples include zinc oxide and titanium dioxide. Both these chemicals are normally used in a micronised form. That means they are very tiny particles of these metal-based ingredients.

Microfine particles are smaller than those used in conventional white zinc sunscreens and are usually in the range of 100–2500 nm (a nanometre, nm, is one millionth of a millimetre). In the process used to manufacture microfine particles, some particles can inadvertently be ground smaller, ending up being classified as nano-sized. Nanoparticles are smaller than 100 nm and invisible to the human eye. There have been concerns that nanoparticles in sunscreens pose a health risk; these concerns will be addressed in detail later.

The advantage of using inorganic UV filters in the extremely tiny form is that it gives them good sun protection properties. They do not leave the skin looking white or leave obvious visible signs of a cream or lotion.

Inorganic chemical filters are sometimes referred to as physical blockers, but this term should be avoided. That is because it may create an expectation of sunscreens blocking the sun's UV rays. They cannot do that. Sunscreen only 'filters' the UV radiation. It is like the difference between a flyscreen door –which lets some things in – compared to a solid door. Sunscreen is more like the flyscreen.

Organic UV filters

The term 'organic' should not be confused with organically grown vegetables, essential oils or other plant-derived ingredients; it simply refers to the fact that the active UV filters contain carbon atoms. Organic chemical absorbers are classified into either UVA or UVB filters depending on the type of radiation they largely absorb. Examples of UVA absorbers that you might read on a sunscreen bottle include oxybenzone and avobenzone, whereas UVB absorbers include salicylates, cinnamates and camphor derivatives.

In most sunscreens, inorganic UV filters are generally combined with organic UV filters to achieve high SPFs.

What wavelengths should sunscreens protect against?

Chapter 2 describes the difference between UVA and UVB, as different parts of the UV spectrum that comes from the sun. In most circumstances, the different parts of the UV spectrum make no difference to how we protect ourselves in the sun. Clothing, hats and shade all protect against UV radiation, whether it is UVA or UVB. The only time it becomes important is in the formulation of the sunscreen we use.

We do not yet fully understand the importance of different wavelengths of UV radiation with regard to long-term effects of sun on the skin such as ageing and skin cancer, especially the serious type of skin cancer known as malignant melanoma. Although the increased diagnosis of malignant melanoma in many countries, not least Australia, has been attributed to changing patterns of sun exposure, the relevant wavelengths of UV in causing this disease remain under

Three girls and three sunscreens

Suppose that three girls – Ann, Betsy and Clare – use sunscreens with the same SPF but with different active UV filters.

- Ann uses a sunscreen that contains active ingredients which absorb mainly UVB radiation. This is typical of sunscreens used in the 1980s and 1990s.
- Betsy uses a product which combines active filters that absorb both UVB and, to a lesser extent, UVA. This is typical of many products that have been on the market for the past 10 years or so.
- Clare uses a sunscreen which is a broad-spectrum sunscreen sold in the past year or two and which provides balanced protection across the UV spectrum.

All the sunscreens have the same SPF rating and the girls all use the same amount of sunscreen.

Each girl is in the sun for the same time but do they all receive the same UV dose? After all, they all use sunscreen with the same SPF rating and so they should be protected equally against sunburn.

The answer is *No*.

Clare is the best protected. Betsy will receive a UV dose to her skin that is 50% more than Clare's, while Ann receives three times the UV dose that Clare does. The moral is: always use a sunscreen offering broad-spectrum protection to minimise the overall UV exposure of your skin.

debate. It would seem sensible, therefore, to use sunscreens that absorb more or less uniformly throughout the UV spectrum, i.e. they absorb both UVB and UVA to much the same extent.

The rationale is that our skin has evolved to exist in harmony with the mix of wavelengths that make up the spectrum of sunlight here on the Earth's surface. Nature understands the importance of this – when we seek natural shade or wear clothing to protect our skin from UV, we reduce the intensity or power of sunlight on our skin but only minimally change the spectrum, or the relative mixture of different wavelengths.

Another benefit of using a broad-spectrum sunscreen is that the total UV dose absorbed by the skin is much less than if a sunscreen of the same SPF is used but it absorbs mainly UVB radiation.

It is now widely accepted that sunscreens should provide balanced, broad-spectrum protection. With these increasing expectations on sunscreen, manufacturers have developed products with spectral profiles that approach this ideal. There has been major improvement in sunscreens over the past 10 years and today there are products that provide excellent broad-spectrum sun protection.

For example, a modern high SPF (30+) broad-spectrum sunscreen might contain the following five active UV filters: octocrylene, bis-ethylhexyloxyphenol methoxyphenyl triazine, butyl methoxydibenzoylmethane, ethylhexyl salicylate and diethylhexyl butamido triazone. This might sound like a complicated and scary chemical soup, but it is important to recognise that a modern, broad-spectrum sunscreen will often contain a variety of chemically complex, effective active UV filters.

The sunscreen–sunburn paradox

There are a lot of reports of sunburn occurring in people using sunscreen. Why might that happen when sunburn prevention is by far the most common reason for using sunscreens, and laboratory testing confirms that sunscreens will prevent erythema (the clinical name for sunburn)?

The SPF required to prevent sunburn can easily be determined if we know the local solar UV levels, the time spent and the behaviour outdoors of someone using sunscreen, and their personal susceptibility to sunburn. Maximum daily UV levels (ambient UV), which occur on the ground, under a completely open (i.e. no shade), cloudless summer sky are ~60–70 SED in Australia and 40–50 SED for Europe. SED stands for standard erythema dose, a measure of the UV dose of sunlight that results in sunburn; it requires an exposure of ~2 SED to produce a very mild sunburn in sun-sensitive individuals who burn easily and never tan. This rises to ~4–5 SED in people with naturally white skin but who tan easily. People with darker or brown skin can still burn but that might require 6 SED or more.

People will not get these maximum ambient exposures because it would be extremely unlikely for someone to lie flat in the unshaded sun all day without moving. An extreme sunbaker might spend half the time lying on their back and half the time face down, resulting in a maximum exposure on much of the body surface of ~50% of total ambient UV. For people who are upright and mobile, engaging in an outdoor pursuit such as gardening, walking or sport, the exposure relative to ambient on commonly exposed sites (e.g. the chest, shoulder, face, forearms and lower legs) ranges from ~5% to 60%, depending on the particular body site and the presence of nearby shade, such as buildings or trees.

So someone in Australia who spends all day sunbaking on a clear summer day with no clothing or other protection would receive a daily skin exposure of no more than 70 SED × 50% = 35 SED. If they have skin that responds typically to sunlight, they would need to use a sunscreen that reduces this exposure to, e.g., 3 SED or less if they are to avoid any skin reddening (i.e. sunburn) that evening. In other words, the sunscreen should provide protection against the amount of UV (35 SED) divided by the target amount of exposure (3 SED) or 12-fold protection. Or put another way, it should have an SPF of 12. If you are walking around in an urban environment, where you may receive ~20% of ambient on exposed sites such as the arms and face, theoretically you should avoid sunburn if you are wearing a product providing an SPF of [70 SED × 20%]/ 3 SED = SPF5.

So, why do people who use high factor (SPF15+) sunscreen experience sunburn so frequently? There are several reasons why their protection is often less than that expected.

Factors affecting the protection provided by sunscreens

There are several factors that determine why most people who use sunscreens receive less protection than they are expecting from the labelled SPF.

- application thickness;
- application technique;
- sunscreen type;
- sunscreen formulation;
- water immersion;
- reapplication.

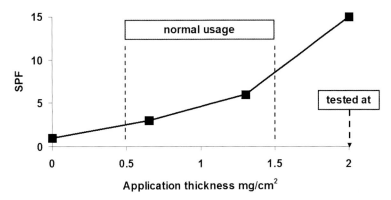

Fig. 5.2: Variation in SPF with applied thickness for a sunscreen labelled SPF15. Note that people applying typical thicknesses of 0.5–1.5 mg/cm² will only receive ~3-fold to 10-fold protection even though they are expecting 15-fold protection.

Application thickness

The protection offered by a sunscreen – defined by its SPF – is assessed after testing a group of volunteers in a laboratory at an internationally agreed application thickness of 2 mg/cm². Yet many studies show that consumers in real-life situations apply much less than this – typically 0.5–1.5 mg/cm², i.e. 25–75% of the amount used by manufacturers in the testing process that determines the SPF number on the container. Figure 5.2 shows how the protection factor of a sunscreen varies with the amount applied. It is clear that most users probably achieve a level of protection 20–50% of that expected from the SPF on the product label.

Application technique

When sunscreens are tested on volunteers in the laboratory to determine their SPF, great care is taken to apply a uniform layer of sunscreen over the test area by spreading with a gloved finger. In practice, of course, nothing like this care is taken when sunscreen is applied to the skin. Sunscreen is normally spread haphazardly and non-uniformly with the result that patchy sunburn may appear after sun exposure (Fig. 5.3).

Spray-on sunscreens have become popular in recent years but, as Fig. 5.4 illustrates, unexpected sunburn can occur if they are not spread carefully over the skin after application.

Even when people decide to use sunscreen, they may not always choose to apply it to all exposed sites. This is illustrated in Fig. 5.5, which summarises the results of asking 100 British adults (51 male) the following question: 'If you decide to use a sunscreen, do you always apply it to each of these sites if they are uncovered?' Fewer than half the people questioned always apply sunscreen

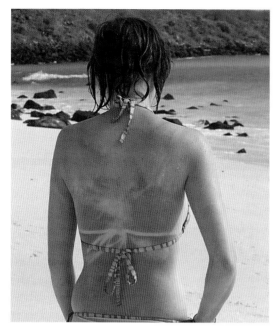

Fig. 5.3: The consequence of non-uniform sunscreen application. Photo courtesy of http://www.philip.greenspun.com.

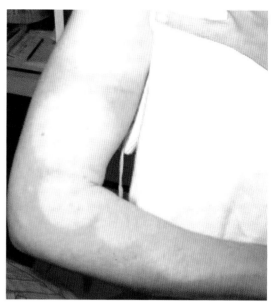

Fig. 5.4: Protected skin within the diameter of the sunscreen spray's mist with surrounding sunburn. Source: Barr (2005). Reproduced with permission.

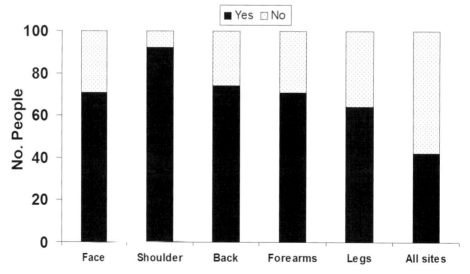

Fig. 5.5: 100 people were asked 'If you decide to use a sunscreen, do you always apply it to each of these sites if they are uncovered?' 71 people said they always applied sunscreen to their face, while 29 people said they didn't always do this, and so on.

to all uncovered sites, even if they decide to use sunscreen. Areas most likely to be missed during sunscreen application are the ears, neck, feet and legs.

Sunscreen type

Sunscreens containing inorganic chemicals, such as zinc oxide or titanium dioxide, as the sole active ingredient can sometimes leave a white film on the skin. As a consequence, people may use less than they would apply if products incorporate organic filters. This can reduce the protection achieved, which is especially unfortunate because some inorganic sunscreens were marketed as 'total sunblocks'. These tended to be used by sun-sensitive individuals, including those with sensitive skin or eczema. The term 'sunblock' can no longer be used to describe sunscreens in Australia. This is because sunscreen never achieves a total sun blocking effect, so the claim is now considered misleading.

Sunscreen formulation

The formulation of the sunscreen can be important in influencing our willingness to use and reapply a sunscreen. Creams have lost popularity as they are less easy to rub into the skin and can leave a white film, which many people find unacceptable. High-SPF products, which could previously be found only in cream formulations, now include lotions, milks, gels, sticks and sprays.

In one study of products designed for use on the face, including lotions, creams, gels and sprays, an alcohol-based spray formulation of sunscreen was rated the most favourable. The alcohol-based sunscreen was said to be less greasy and less likely to leave a film than at least two of the other sunscreens evaluated.

The importance of good formulation, resulting in a cosmetically appealing product, is increasingly recognised by manufacturers. It is all very well making a sunscreen with a very high SPF but if consumers don't like the feel or look of it, they won't use it. Or people may apply so little that the real protection they are getting leaves them vulnerable to sunburn and skin damage. Figure 5.6 compares two sunscreens, one with a formulation that results in a colourless film on the skin and the other that tends to leave a white residue. Most people seem to prefer avoiding the appearance of visible sunscreen on their skin.

When you are choosing a sunscreen, try to test a small amount on the back of your hand first before buying it to get an idea of whether you'll like putting it on your skin. And keep using it! Remember, it's not all about the SPF.

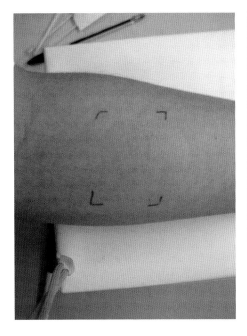
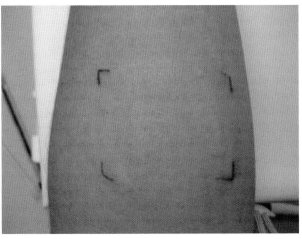

Fig. 5.6: The sunscreen on the left leaves an invisible film on the skin, while that on the right leaves a white residue.

Water immersion

Many people love swimming, bathing and water sports – and generally more skin is exposed to the sun while doing so. It is an obvious time for people to use sunscreen. This has led to the development of products that bind well to the skin surface and resist washing-off. So much so that the majority of sunscreen products now available for recreational use claim to be 'water-resistant'.

Sunscreens in Australia are no longer allowed to claim to be 'waterproof'. Like the concerns over the use of the word 'sunblock', claims of being waterproof are beyond what sunscreen can usually achieve and so are now considered misleading.

The change in measured SPF for two products both claiming SPF15 following four 20-minute immersions of volunteers in water is shown in Figure 5.7. The sunscreen claiming water resistance showed a small gradual decrease in protection over four immersions. The product designed for daily skincare that contained UV filters but made no claims concerning water resistance, lost most of its sun protection properties after just one immersion. If you apply a facial moisturiser that contains UV filters (as most moisturisers do these days) in the morning and wash your face before lunchtime, you'll have lost any UV protection before you go outside at midday.

It remains true that the most common activity during which Australians experience sunburn involves water. Whether at the beach, the pool or other water-based activity, using water-resistant sunscreen clearly makes sense.

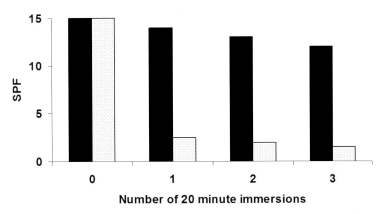

Fig. 5.7: The change in SPF with water immersion for a sunscreen claiming to be waterproof (solid block) and a day-care product that made no claim concerning water resistance (shaded area).

Reapplication

The main reason for reapplying sunscreen during sun exposure is to compensate for initial under-application so as to achieve an SPF more in line with the rated value. Another reason is to replace sunscreen that may have been removed by water, vigorous towelling or friction with clothing or sand. Inadequate application is the primary purpose for reapplication since modern water-resistant sunscreens adhere well to the surface of the skin, even after immersion in water.

Guidance on sunscreen packs about reapplication is generally to 'reapply frequently' or 'reapply regularly' and a common recommendation by the Cancer Council is to reapply sunscreen every two hours. Maybe because of cost, or just forgetting, it seems not many users reapply sunscreens frequently or regularly.

If you use a sunscreen that is easily removed from the skin then you will achieve little in the way of sun protection, no matter when it is reapplied. Better sun protection will be achieved with a reapplication of sunscreen ~20–30 minutes after being in the sun, rather than waiting two to three hours, after initial application. Reapplication of sunscreen 20 minutes into a four-hour exposure period to summer sunshine results in 50–75% of the UV exposure that would be received, compared with waiting two hours before the sunscreen is reapplied.

People are advised to apply sunscreen liberally or generously. However, many studies have shown that users feel uncomfortable with application at 2 mg/cm^2 – the thickness used by manufacturers during the testing process to determine the SPF. Generally people prefer to apply quantities of about half this thickness. That people generally apply less than 2 mg/cm^2 has led many commentators into the trap of believing that consumers use inadequate amounts of sunscreen for protection. There is another way to look at this problem. It could be argued that people use the quantity they feel comfortable with and in this sense are using the 'correct' amount; it is the labelled SPFs, driven by the testing system, that could be considered misleading.

How much is enough ? To achieve the level of sun protection as claimed by the SPF on the container, the average adult wearing little clothing (e.g. 'speedos' on men and bikinis on women) would need to apply ~35 mL of sunscreen. That would amount to about seven teaspoons (~5 mL per teaspoon) of sunscreen on their body, i.e. about one teaspoon per limb, one on the front and one on the back of the torso and one on the face and neck. But very few people take a teaspoon to the beach!

While sunscreen is sold in containers of many shapes and sizes, the 110 mL tube is a common size. A single application of 35 mL would be about one-third of a 110 mL tube. Human nature being what it is, there are abundant data to show that most people don't use this quantity of sunscreen at each application and it is likely, therefore, that campaigns to encourage people to use a greater quantity of sunscreen for a single application will fail.

An important factor in sunscreen performance is the uneven nature of the skin surface. If an opaque sunscreen is applied to the skin, the surface markings become visible as the grooves on the skin surface are filled. With further application, the intervening ridges are also covered and the surface becomes more featureless. The situation is a little like painting a wall with a textured surface (see Fig. 5.8) – two coats of paint are almost always needed for satisfactory coverage. In the same way, two coats of sunscreen may be required for adequate protection.

When thinking about the amount of protection sunscreen can offer, it is important to understand that a second application does not 'restart the clock' when estimating the amount of

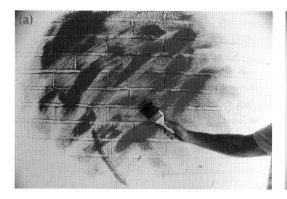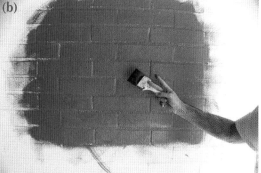

Fig. 5.8: Like painting a wall with a textured surface, two coats of sunscreen may be required for adequate protection to the textured skin surface.

time that we can safely spend in the sun. Whether applied 20 minutes or two hours after the first application, the amount of time skin is protected must start from when sun exposure started. There is always some UV that reaches the skin no matter how much sunscreen is applied to the skin. The reapplication is primarily to ensure the best possible protection is delivered as a result of more uniform and substantial application. It does not erase the UV exposure that has already occurred before the second layer of sunscreen is applied.

Reapplying sunscreen early into your sun exposure period may well be more successful than doing so two hours in, when you are more likely forget. Tips for applying sunscreen are as follows.

- Apply sunscreen liberally to exposed sites 15–30 minutes before going out into the sun.
- Don't rub the sunscreen into your skin. Spread it as uniformly as possible over the surface of the skin and allow it to dry.
- Reapply sunscreen to exposed sites 15–30 minutes after sun exposure begins.
- Further reapplication of sunscreen is necessary after vigorous activity that could remove sunscreen, such as swimming, towelling, excessive sweating and rubbing.

All the factors described above mean that, as a rule of thumb, the protection achieved from applying a sunscreen is estimated as typically about half to one-third of the rated SPF. So in order to achieve 10–15-fold protection, a sunscreen rated at least SPF30+ needs to be applied.

Finally, don't forget that people tend to apply sunscreen more frequently on summer days when the weather is fine and they intend spending recreational time outdoors. And it is on days such as these that they are most vulnerable to sunburn if sunscreen application is less than ideal.

Are sunscreens safe?

Expert reviews of sunscreen safety and efficacy conclude that the current list of commonly used organic and inorganic active ingredients do not pose a concern for human health. However, although it's uncommon, sunscreens occasionally cause skin irritation or a skin allergy. Nevertheless, concern about any adverse effects of using sunscreen continues to generate interest.

Endocrine disruption

Reports of oestrogenic effects of some UV filters have given rise to concern that applying sunscreen may prove a risk to human health. Oestrogen is the female sex hormone that controls a range of important bodily functions. Several studies have suggested a weak oestrogenic activity of several UV filters in lab tests. However, this weak activity does not appear to have an effect in people. In a careful assessment of the most potent UV filters with oestrogen-like activity, 3-(4-methyl benzylidene) camphor, the Scientific Committee on Consumer Products in Europe concluded that there was no risk to humans. There is little convincing evidence linking sunscreen use to endocrine-disruptive effects in humans.

Vitamin D deficiency

The issue of vitamin D is addressed in detail in Chapter 8. Sunlight produces vitamin D in the skin, necessary for strong healthy bones. It has been suggested that current sun avoidance practices including the use of sunscreens may contribute to vitamin D deficiency. This is supported by laboratory studies which show that application of sunscreen will reduce artificial UV-induced vitamin D in people.

Yet studies examining vitamin D status in prospective human studies of sunscreen use have not found deficiencies in vitamin D. This is probably because of the haphazard nature of sunscreen application and the fact that some exposed sites will often be left unprotected, as illustrated in Fig. 5.5.

Nanoparticles

Increasingly, sunscreen manufacturers are using very tiny particles as active ingredients in sunscreen. Earlier, we discussed microfine particles and the fact that in the manufacturing process used to produce microfine particles, some particles can inadvertently be ground smaller, ending up as nanoparticles.

Based on current evidence, the risk to humans from the use of nano-structured titanium dioxide or zinc oxide in sunscreens was considered negligible in a 2010 report by an expert review panel. The panel found that the micronised and nano-structured UV filters can be regarded as safe for use at the concentrations found in sunscreen products.

All sunscreens in Australia are tightly regulated through the Therapeutic Goods Administration (TGA). In 2009, the TGA conducted an updated review of the scientific literature in relation to the use of nano-structured zinc oxide and titanium dioxide in sunscreens. The TGA review concluded that the potential for these two molecules in sunscreens to cause harmful effects depends on the ability of the nanoparticles to reach living skin cells. So far the evidence suggests that titanium dioxide and zinc oxide in micronised form do not damage these vulnerable skin cells.

Regardless of the best available evidence, there will continue to be questions as 'nano' conjures up images of technology gone awry. Yet the overwhelming expert view is that the public health benefits of sunscreens containing micronised (nano) titanium dioxide or zinc oxide outweigh human safety concerns for these UV filters.

Is it safe to use sunscreen on babies?

You're at the beach applying your sunscreen. Your five-month-old baby is there with you, so should you put sunscreen on him/her? This is best avoided in infants less than six months of age as babies' skin is thinner than that of adults and it can absorb the UV active chemical ingredients in sunscreen more easily. Also, infants have a high surface-area to bodyweight ratio compared to older children and adults. Both these factors mean that a baby's exposure to the chemicals in sunscreens is greater, increasing the risk of an allergic reaction.

The best approach is to keep infants under six months out of direct sun and in the shade as much as possible. This is especially important around the middle of the day when UV rays are most intense. Make sure your child wears loose-fitting clothing that covers the skin and keeps them cool – and don't forget a sunhat! If there's no way to keep your baby out of the sun, you can apply a small amount of high SPF sunscreen to small areas such as the cheeks and back of the hands.

How long will sunscreens keep?

Sunscreens are emulsions of oil and water and so will tend to separate. The time this takes depends on the quality of the formulation; it can vary from a few months to many years or even decades. Typically, the shelf life of sunscreens is 30 months.

To maximise their quality, sunscreens should be stored in a cool dry place, out of direct sunlight. If you are concerned about your sunscreen, have a smell and feel of the product – if it seems okay and has been stored correctly, it should be fine to use. However, as a final check you should refer to the 'use by date' on the labelling, as products do have a fixed life after they have been opened.

Finally, there is the question of microbiological integrity once the sunscreen has been opened and used for the first time. This tends to shorten its physical stability, particularly these days when allergy concerns have led to the minimal use of preservatives in sunscreens.

Is there evidence that sunscreens prevent skin cancer?

Knowledge of the harmful effects of sunlight has increased dramatically in the past two decades, largely due to the combined efforts of public health agencies and the media. People are now much more aware of the risk of skin cancer, which is the most common human cancer – over 2 million people worldwide each year get skin cancer. People apply sunscreens in the belief that doing so will reduce this risk. So what evidence is there that sunscreens are effective in this important public health arena?

Sunscreen use and prevention of non-melanoma skin cancer

The strongest available evidence that sunscreen use is an effective approach to prevention of non-melanoma skin cancers, which account for ~90% of all skin cancers and include basal cell cancer (BCC) and squamous cell cancer (SCC), comes from the results of a community-based trial in which 1621 adults aged 25–75 were randomly selected from all residents of Nambour, a subtropical Queensland township ~100 km north of Brisbane.

Trial participants were randomised either to apply a freely supplied broad-spectrum sunscreen with an SPF16 daily to the head and arms for 4.5 years, or to continue their usual level of sunscreen use or non-use. In comparison with people not asked to use sunscreen on a daily basis, the treatment group showed a 40% reduction in SCC tumours at the conclusion of the trial. Eight years after the study, participants who had been asked to use daily sunscreen continued to show a 40% decrease in SCC incidence.

Although there was no effect on BCC incidence during the trial period, there was a trend of increasing intervals between BCCs among the sunscreen-using group compared with people in the control group who developed multiple BCCs.

Sunscreen use and prevention of melanoma

The observation that sunscreens protect against sunburn led to the common expectation that they will also protect against skin cancer, including malignant melanoma. Despite this commonly held perception, the scientific evidence that sunscreen prevents melanoma remains controversial.

It is not surprising that studies looking at the link between sunscreen use and melanoma risk are inconclusive. It is known that people more likely to use sunscreen (because they have sun-sensitive skin) are also at higher risk of melanoma. So we might expect people diagnosed with melanoma to report using sunscreen more commonly than people who tolerate sunlight well and are at lower risk of melanoma. Also, the sunscreens available during the period relevant to these studies were generally of a much lower standard than those that are now available. They were particularly less effective in protecting against UVA and people tended to use products with much lower SPFs than they do today. The tendency for people to use less sunscreen than required to achieve the labelled protection is another reason why the studies found little melanoma protection.

To date, there is one important finding that suggests that sunscreens may have a role to play in preventing melanoma. Ten years after the end of the sunscreen intervention trial in Nambour, the group of 812 people who were asked to use daily sunscreen had experienced 11 new melanomas, compared with the control group of 809, who experienced 22 new melanomas. While the number of melanomas in the daily sunscreen group was half the number appearing in the control group, the small number of melanomas recorded to that point in the study means that the result is still 'early days'. Further evidence that sunscreens really do prevent melanoma is badly needed.

Sunscreens, melanoma and the precautionary principle

We have, then, a dilemma. Applying the principles of evidence-based medicine, there is not yet strong enough evidence to use sunscreens as a preventative measure in melanoma. And gathering evidence on whether modern, high-SPF broad-spectrum sunscreens are effective would take a decade or more. Because of the limited body of evidence, some would argue that the focus of recommendations for melanoma prevention in public health campaigns should be more on sun avoidance, shade and clothing.

On the other hand there is the precautionary principle, which states that if an action or policy might cause severe or irreversible harm to the public then, in the absence of a scientific consensus that harm would not ensue, the burden of proof falls on people who would advocate taking the action. In other words, those who say that sunscreens should not be used as a preventative measure in melanoma because of limited evidence for their efficacy must demonstrate that lack of efficacy for their advice to be followed. Logic would suggest that demonstrating lack of efficacy would be difficult, as exposure to UV radiation is widely recognised as a risk factor in melanoma and modern sunscreens attenuate the intensity of solar UV entering the skin.

Conclusion

Applying sunscreen is just one element of a strategy aimed at controlling sun exposure, which includes seeking shade, avoiding the sun around the middle of the day and wearing clothing and wide-brimmed hats. Sunscreen application can be problematic. The amount normally applied is insufficient to achieve the rated SPF, and that which is applied is often spread non-uniformly. This often results in some exposed skin sites achieving little or no protection. In addition, sunscreen is removed to a greater or lesser extent due to activities such as swimming and towelling, and reapplication often takes place when the skin has already been exposed to sufficient sunlight to result in sunburn.

These factors, coupled with other factors discussed above, provide ample evidence that the numerical measure of protection indicated on the product pack by the SPF is generally higher than that achieved in real life. This mismatch between expectation and reality may be one contributing factor why sunscreens have not yet been conclusively confirmed to prevent melanoma. For this reason, sunscreen should not be considered the first line of defence against excessive sun exposure.

On the other hand, debate over the efficacy of sunscreens should not prevent their use, alongside other sun protective measures, during recreational summer sun exposure. The corollary to this advice is, of course, that their use must not lead to deliberately excessive sun exposure – inadequate and non-uniform application, coupled with extended times in the sun, could result in unacceptably high exposure of 'sunscreen-protected' skin.

Further reading

Barr J (2005) Spray-on sunscreens need a good rub. *Journal of the American Academy of Dermatology* **52**, 180–181. doi:10.1111/j.1600-0781.2009.00459.x.

Diffey BL (2009) Sunscreens: expectation and realisation. *Photodermatology, Photoimmunology and Photomedicine* **25**, 233–236. doi:10.1111/j.1600-0781.2009.00459.x.

Green AC, Williams GM, Logan V, Strutton GM (2011) Reduced melanoma after regular sunscreen use: randomized trial follow-up. *Journal of Clinical Oncology* **29**, 257–263. doi:10.1200/JCO.2010.28.7078.

IARC (2000) Handbooks of Cancer Prevention. Vol. 5, *Sunscreens*. International Agency for Research on Cancer, Lyon.

Lim HW, Draelos ZD (eds) (2009) *A Clinical Guide to Sunscreens and Photoprotection*. Informa Healthcare USA, New York.

Nash JF (2006) Human safety and efficacy of ultraviolet filters and sunscreen products. *Dermatologic Clinics* **24**, 35–51. doi:10.1016/j.det.2005.09.006.

Therapeutic Goods Administration (2009) *A Review of the Scientific Literature on the Safety of Nanoparticulate Titanium Dioxide or Zinc Oxide in Sunscreens.* Commonwealth Department of Health and Ageing. Available at http://www.tga.gov.au/pdf/sunscreens-nanoparticles-2009.pdf (accessed 28 June 2013).

Chapter 6

'Seek shade': have it made in the shade

Christina Mackay

Key messages

- The use of shade has a long history in Australia and New Zealand as a means of reducing the impact of our intense sunshine.
- The way we choose to build in and modify our natural environment must consider the need for the right shade in the right place using the right design. It differs from the needs of many of our forebears, who immigrated from cooler climates.
- An issue often ignored is the importance of diffuse UV, the UV radiation (UVR) that is scattered in the atmosphere, as compared to the direct UV which reaches us in sunshine.
- In open-sky situations, without buildings or natural features like trees, diffuse UV can contribute up to half of our total UV exposure so we need to design ways to protect ourselves from it.
- Good shade design, and careful choice of materials and planting, can cool or warm outdoor spaces to create safe and comfortable environments year-round as well as helping to control our UVR exposure.
- Correct design using the correct material with an understanding of the local environment are all essential ingredients in getting shade right.

Introduction

Six months ago, my 50-year-old brother, a fourth-generation New Zealander with Scottish ancestry, had a melanoma removed. Although now living in Singapore, he had spent his childhood on a farm, his student years windsurfing and later he lived close to the sea enjoying beach culture. Thankfully, the malignant cells had not spread. I recently asked him how this event had changed his lifestyle. He said the change was dramatic and he now 'walked in the shade'. He completely avoided the direct sun but was concerned that he would not get enough UVR exposure and might suffer from vitamin D deficiency. In this chapter, my aim is to share my view on why his UVR overexposure happened, explain the architectural science of shading from UVR and show how he (and all fair-skinned Australasians) can create a 'shady' lifestyle both for themselves and their descendants.

First, I will explain why shade for UVR is important for many Australasians, and how our cultural heritage of building and landscape design and patterns of lifestyle influence our relation to sunshine.

Australasia has a unique challenge

When presenting research on UVR protective shade at architectural conferences around the world, the subject was new to the audiences. In Chile, the majority of the population are darker-skinned and prevention campaigns for other cancers were considered of higher priority. In Canada and the northern states of the USA, the audiences were bemused. In Seattle, locals soaked up every ray of sunshine. The summers there are short with maximum estimated UVR level of UVI 8. In northern Europe, summers are also short, but many Europeans and the British get sunburned during brief sun-filled holidays on the Mediterranean coast or further afield. Protecting themselves from the sun on an everyday basis was not a high concern.

In Australia and New Zealand, fair-skinned populations have settled in lands with very high UVR levels and clear skies. This environment is not their genetic homeland. The dark skin of the indigenous Australians evolved over thousands of years to provide protection for their traditional hunter–gatherer lifestyle in the large open plentiful continent. The hot climate necessitated few clothes and simple shade canopies to shelter from the heat of the sun.

Shade ancestry

For fair-skinned Australasians, the challenge is to use natural and built environments to create a shady lifestyle for themselves and future generations. The issue is not a temporary one. The skins

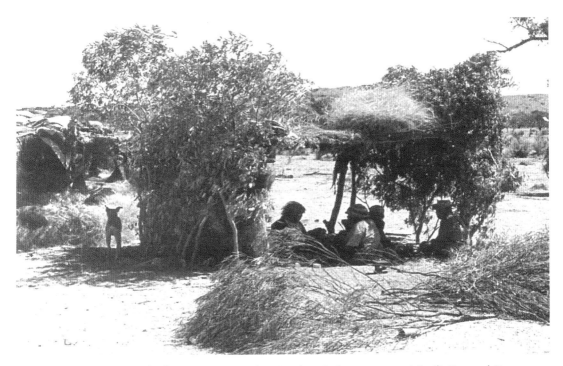

Fig. 6.1: This day-time shade structure was in a Yankuntjatjara camp at Mimili, Everard Ranges, South Australia 1970. Source: Annette Hamilton.

of future Australasians may well darken with intermarriage and the very slow process of genetic evolution, but if it happens this will take hundreds or thousands of years. The evolution of creating UVR-protective living environments is a faster approach.

To find design solutions, we can learn from peoples who have lived with high sunshine levels for millennia. Indigenous Australians designed structures to shade from the heat of the sun (Fig. 6.1). A common form was a low rectangular post and beam structure with the top and some sides covered in tree branches.

This shade shelter was effective in creating a cooler space as well as shielding from UVR. While the surrounding trees had sparse leaves, the layering of the branches created a dense barrier to direct sunshine (including UVR). The low square roof was a good shield to high midday sun. The vegetation on the sides shielded morning and afternoon direct sun. Under the shade, it appears that little open sky would be in view through the two openings. This is important as the open sky reflects diffuse UV.

In tropical northern Australia, where there is ample water, tree canopies are very dense and shield direct UV well. These trees, in the process of evapotranspiration, release water vapour into the air.

This process can cool the air temperature by 2–3°C. In wet tropical or subtropical areas, green landscape can provide excellent outdoor shade. In hot arid zones, it is often necessary to build shade.

For many generations, families have emigrated from countries around the Mediterranean. The olive skins of their ancestors evolved to suit the sunny climate, as did the design of their houses and townscapes. Houses with thick stone walls and terracotta tiled roofs created a barrier to the hot sun and kept the interiors cool. Exterior window shutters shielded the direct sun but allowed cooling breezes. The tall narrow streets usually created a shady side on which to walk and a small view of the sky. A paved open square would absorb the hot midday sun while the villagers were indoors enjoying their siesta. This heat was released in the cool of the evening when locals gathered to socialise. These patterns of life evolved to maximise human comfort.

In Italy, villas evolved to include loggia, wide open-sided extensions to houses that provided excellent protection from UVR (Fig. 6.2).

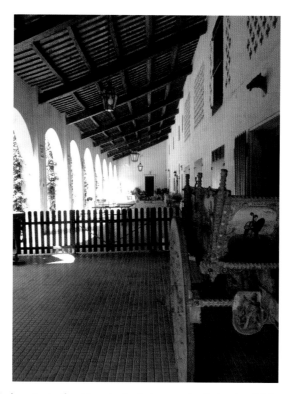

Fig. 6.2: This 5 m wide loggia in the Veneto in Italy was built in the 16th century for farming activities. In the 21st century, it creates a generous outdoor play space for children and family activities. The solid roof is a 100% barrier to direct UV and the garden trees filter diffuse UV. Shaded from the sun, the brick walls and paving radiate cool. © Author.

The ancestors of fair-skinned (skin types 1 + 2, see Fig. 1.7, p. 21) Australians are most likely to have immigrated from the UK, northern Europe and Scandinavia where the summer maximum UVR levels may reach only UVI 5 or 6. There, houses were built without verandas or eaves so the windows could welcome every ray of sunshine. The homes of the first Australian settlers were in this style; later, verandas were added. The word 'veranda' is of Hindi origin. In hot climates, a veranda serves several functions. When the sun is high, it creates a cool space shielded from the direct sun and open to breezes. It also shades the floors and walls, keeping the surfaces cool. In cooler southern climates, the low winter sun floods into a north-facing veranda. In the tropics, where the direct sun is never required for its heat, shutters and louvres are added to shield all sun.

By the early 20th century, verandas were a feature of villas and bungalows in new suburbs. The edges of houses were shady but the suburban streets were wide and open. In Europe in the 1920s, the ancient Greek practice of heliotherapy (using sunlight as a form of disease treatment) was hailed as beneficial for the treatment of tuberculosis and Coco Chanel championed the suntan. This new attitude to the sun was reflected in new architectural fashions. Le Corbusier, the French modernist architect, recommended spaces for sunbathing and designed open sun terraces with large sliding glazed doors from living spaces. Australasian modernist houses followed these trends and promoted large openings onto sun terraces (Fig. 6.3).

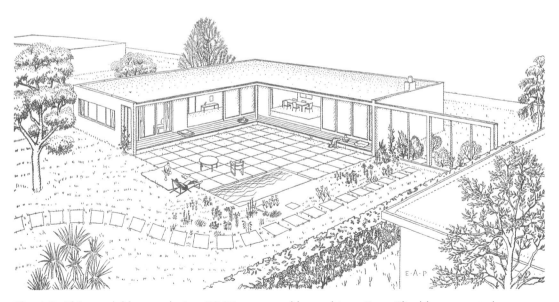

Fig. 6.3: This model house design (1947) proposed by architect Ernst Plischke promoted a sun terrace. The large sliding doors allowed the living room to become open to the outdoors and act as a shady veranda in summer. Source: Plischke (1947).

In the 1980s, when the consequences of sun-worshipping were recognised in terms of high skin cancer rates, along with sun hats and sunscreen, cancer organisations promoted the creation of more shade for our built environment. However, shade was associated with temporary beach umbrellas and fabric sails. Over time many shades became damaged and vandalised, particularly in school grounds. In 2013, permanent COLA (covered outdoor learning areas) for schools were promoted. The COLA initiative acknowledged that 'seeking shade' will be an ongoing necessity for generations of fair-skinned Australians. This requires a permanent change in outdoor living environments.

Shading principles

This section will give you a practical way of evaluating UVR levels in outdoor spaces and strategies for making shade. Understanding how to avoid UVR overexposure comes from careful observation of our everyday environment and lifestyle patterns. To design effective outdoor shaded space, you need to understand how different skin types react to the sun, the seasonal and daily patterns of UVR intensity for your geographical location and how UV exposure comprises direct, diffuse and reflected UVR. To shield the direct sun, you need to locate seasonal daily sun-paths and choose the shading material carefully. Finally, outdoor areas need to be thermally and visually comfortable if they are going to be used. The overall design and use of different materials can modify the climate significantly.

Skin type

It is important to understand the skin type of you and your family and the time it takes for the first signs of sunburn to occur at different UVR intensities. Figure 6.4 illustrates this in relation to UVI.

Seasonal and daily UV levels

Chapter 2 presented coloured charts (Fig. 2.12, p. 44) illustrating daily UVR levels throughout the year in different locations around Australia. These charts are most useful in determining when it is necessary to avoid direct sunshine. It is important to remember that the UVI levels are an estimation of the maximum potential hazard on a cloudless day in an open location (equivalent to a flat plain). Hills, trees and buildings can reduce UVR exposure significantly by shielding diffuse UVR as described in the following section.

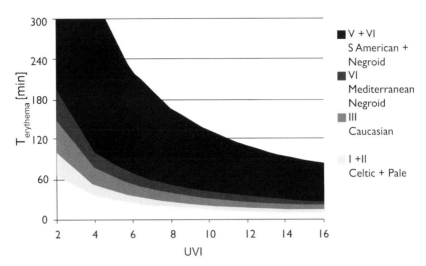

Fig. 6.4: This graph illustrates how different skin types (as defined by Fitzpatrick in 1988) react to increasing intensities of UVR. $T_{erythema}$ is the time (in minutes) it takes for the first signs of sunburn to appear.

Direct and diffuse UV

We receive UVR from two main sources outdoors. Direct UVR is radiated directly from the sun, in sunshine. Diffuse UVR is reflected from the hemisphere of the atmosphere above, the visible sky. When the sun is high we receive slightly more direct UVR than indirect UVR, and when the sun is low we receive slightly less direct UVR than indirect UVR. However, in designing shade it is useful to consider that in an open field situation a person will receive on average ~50% of UV from the direct sun and ~50% from UV reflected from the hemisphere.

For practical purposes, the diffuse UV can be considered to be equally distributed around the hemisphere. So if the UVI level is predicted to be UVI 10, it could be predicted that a person would receive approximately UVI 5 from the direct sun and UVI 5 from diffuse UV reflected from the hemisphere of the open sky (Fig. 6.5).

The amount of UVR exposure of a person standing in the shade can be estimated by observing the solidness of the shading material and the proportion of the sky hemisphere that can be seen. For example, consider a person standing in the shadow of a wall on a flat plain (Fig. 6.6). They are receiving no direct sun and can see only approximately half the hemisphere of the sky, so if the UVI in the open is UVI 10 then they will be exposed to approximately half the diffuse UVR (UVI 5), i.e. UVI 2.5.

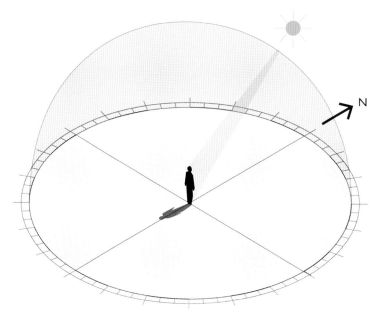

Fig. 6.5: In an open landscape a person will receive ~50% UV exposure from direct sunshine and ~50% from diffuse UV reflected from the hemisphere of open sky.

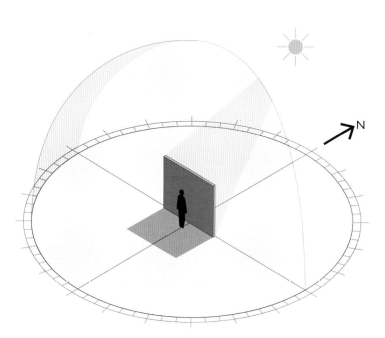

Fig. 6.6: A person standing in the shadow of a wall will receive approximately half the hemisphere of diffuse UV only.

Protection factor (PF) is a concept used to describe the UVR protection provided by fabric or sunscreen (see Chapters 4 and 5). In the same way, the shade provided by the wall is reducing UV exposure by four times (UVI 10 to UVI 2.5) and could be considered to have a protection factor of PF4.

This example illustrates why my brother's strategy of choosing to walk in the shade for short walks is an effective strategy for daily life. (At UVI 2.5 at fair-skinned person will receive the first signs of sunburn in just under an hour.)

Living in a city and urban environments such as downtown Melbourne or Sydney can provide even more protection from diffuse UV. Verandas and tall buildings can significantly reduce the view of the sky (and therefore exposure to diffuse UV).

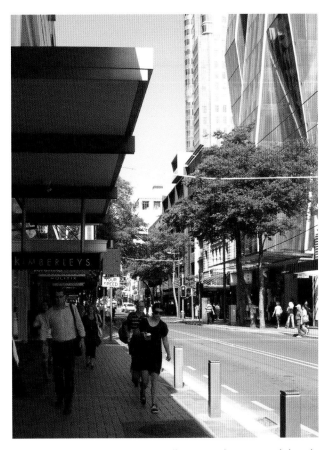

Fig. 6.7: In this view of Willis St in downtown Wellington, the view of the sky could be roughly estimated at 1/5 of the potential sky hemisphere. At UVI 10, a person in the street shade would be exposed to 1/5 diffuse UV = 1/5 × UVI 5 = UVI 1.

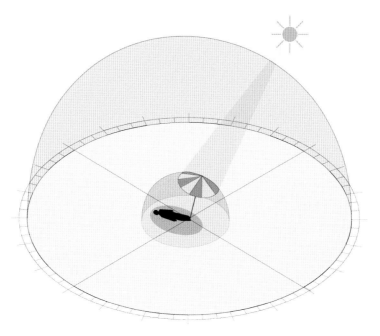

Fig. 6.8: In an open situation, a beach umbrella might shield direct UVR but it provides little protection from diffuse UVR.

Conversely, diffuse UVR can seriously undermine the protection given by an umbrella. Consider a person reading a book under an umbrella in an open landscape (Fig. 6.8). It is an activity that you might enjoy for an hour or two.

By calculating the surface area of the umbrella as a proportion of the hemisphere of the visible sky, a 1600 mm diameter umbrella would shield only 13% of the diffuse UV. If the UV in the open was UVI 10 and the material of the umbrella blocked 95% of UV, the UVR exposure under the shade would be UVI 4.7. A fair-skinned person would experience sunburning in less than 30 minutes. In this example, while the umbrella fabric had a UPF of 20 (the fabric blocks 95% of UVR), the PF of the umbrella canopy was only PF 2.1 (UVI 10 ÷ 4.7).

If the umbrella were situated on a beach, the effective UVI level underneath would be even higher due to the reflected UV off the sand.

Reflected UVR

Generally most materials in the natural world absorb UVR. The darker the material the more the UVR is absorbed, in the same way as a dark-painted wall absorbs the heat of the sun. A grass playground could have 2–5% reflectivity. The reflectivity of new concrete could be 12%, it is only 8% when it is aged. Dry sand can reflect up to 18%. A light-coloured wall would reflect heat, light and UV. At these levels, reflected UV is unlikely to significantly affect the protection factor of a shade canopy in the home environment.

Reflected UVR is critical to consider in outdoor recreational areas, especially in the ski-fields. In these settings you would need to be well protected with clothing and sunscreen.

Sun paths

To make the design of shade structures even more complicated, it is important to understand the different paths of the sun throughout the year. Sun paths for different locations vary accordingly to the movement of the sun around the Earth. Figure 6.9 illustrates the seasonal variation in Tasmania.

Detailed sun-path charts for different locations in Australia are available from various websites and mobile phone apps. Most architectural drawing software can plot building and canopy shadows for any geographical location throughout the day and the year.

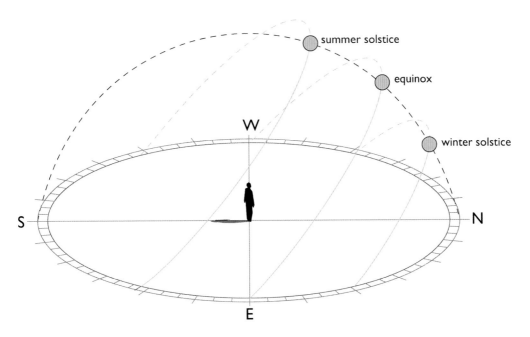

Fig. 6.9: The seasonal sun paths at 42°latitude in Tasmania. In the tropics the sun paths are more directly overhead and there is little seasonal variation.

The aim of good sun protection is to shield the direct sun when UV levels are above UVI 2. While diffuse UV is relatively constant, the angle of direct sunshine is constantly changing both vertically and horizontally.

Screening UV

Shading materials need to be chosen with care, as people can assume that all shade is the same. Solid materials provide a 100% UV barrier; for perforated materials, the percentage is proportional to the solid area (Fig. 6.10).

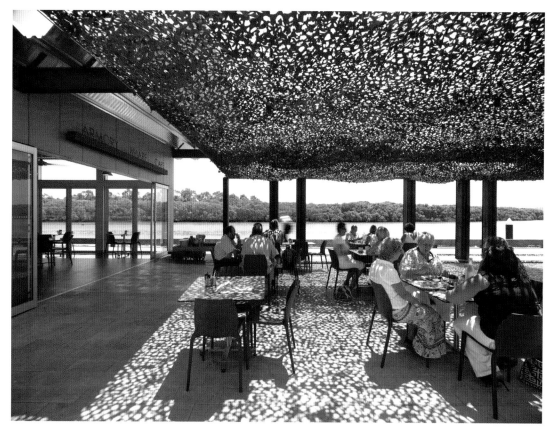

Fig. 6.10: This interesting dappled shade canopy at the Armoury Wharf Café, Sydney (by Lahznimmo Architects) uses army camouflage netting. If the fabric is 50% open, diners would receive ~50% of the outside UVR exposure. At a midsummer lunch-hour in Sydney, the UVR could be UVI 12. Therefore, the effective UVI under the shade could be expected to be UVI 6. Additional sun protection (or moving indoors) would be advisable at this time. © Brett Boardman.

Fabrics provide varying degrees of protection. Generally, dark colours absorb more UVR and therefore create a slightly better barrier (see Chapter 4, p. 67). Horticultural shadecloth offers poor protection. Before selecting any material, it is important to check the manufacturer's specifications for UVR transmission (see Chapter 4 for labelling standards).

Solid materials such as metal, wood or clay roof tiles block UVR 100%. Normal glass filters only part of the UVR erythemal range, but the interlayer of laminated glass (used in overhead glazing and car windscreens) can be a 99% barrier. As UVR degrades most materials, coatings used to protect the base material can protect people as well. The coating on polycarbonate sheeting does this. Some uncoated clear PVCs offer little protection (and break down quickly). ETFE (ethylene tetrafluoroethylene) translucent film has been used to cover sports stadiums. This material transmits a high percentage of UVR, allowing grass underneath to grow. In summary, if you are considering using transparent or translucent shading materials you need to check the technical specifications carefully. Transparent roofing can be appealing as it gives UVR protection that is light and warm.

Green landscaping can also be designed to shield outdoor living spaces. Dense tree canopies provide the best barrier to direct UVR. Outdoor 'walls' of hedges or trellis covered in vines can shield diffuse UVR. In more temperate zones, deciduous trees or vines can allow the low UVR winter sun in, to warm the surrounding surfaces and the occupants. Local advice will help you select the most suitable trees and plants for different climates.

Thermal comfort

In New Zealand and Tasmania, there are times when the air temperature is too cool for comfort but the UVR levels are above UVI 2. In this situation, solid dark shade would be cold and people would not use it. Transparent roofing, together with screening of cool sea breezes, can create a safe and warm outdoor living space. In high summer, fabric or timber screens can be placed under the translucent roofing to shield the radiant heat from the sun.

In other states, people want their outdoor living spaces to be cool. The natural vegetation or bark used as a shading material by Aborigines may have been the most readily available material and was excellent in creating cool shade. It is a barrier to the hot sun and permits cooling breezes. Wooden 'Queenslander' houses (with wide verandas and set high off the ground) are cool for similar reasons. If solid dense materials, such as concrete or stone, can be shaded from the sun, then they stay cool (Fig. 6.11). In contrast, corrugated metal roofing conducts the heat of sun and radiates it to those underneath.

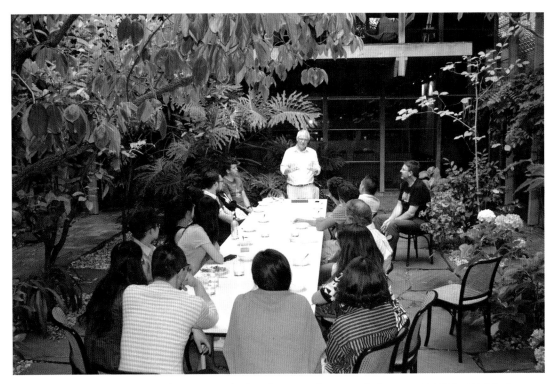

Fig. 6.11: In summer, the leafy courtyard of architect Robin Boyd's house (1958) in Walsh Street, South Yarra, Melbourne creates a cooling microclimate. The trees shade both the people and the surrounding materials. The paving cooled by the night air radiates cool during the day. Evapotranspiration further cools the air. By permission Robin Boyd Foundation.

Wind-loading: permanent versus temporary

Buildings are built to withstand high wind loads. This requires engineered foundations, structural elements and connections and it usually involves considerable expense. In domestic situations, temporary lightweight shadesails and umbrellas can work well. They can be simply taken down if strong winds are forecast. In public and community situations this monitoring is difficult and permanent solutions are better.

Safe and comfortable outdoor environments

Good shade design brings all aspects together. A fine example is the 2001 pavilion in the grounds of Government House in Brisbane, designed by Andresen O'Gorman Architects (Fig. 6.12).

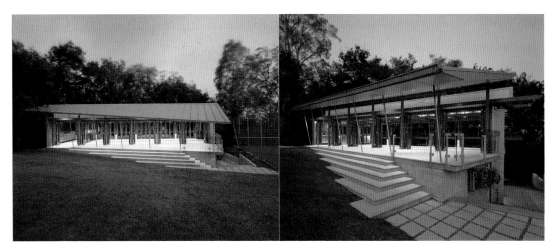

Fig. 6.12: The pavilion (2001) in the grounds of Government House, Brisbane. © Stefan Jannides.

The pavilion is used for community functions which last for two to three hours. As visitors may not be prepared with hats, clothing and sunscreen, the pavilion design was required to give a high level of UV protection. On two sides, the pavilion is nestled into a eucalypt forest shielding diffuse UV from the sky. On this side, translucent roofing allows daylight but is a barrier to UVR. As a person might 'tip their hat' to the sun, a second solid roof slopes downwards to the open lawn, minimising the penetration of both the direct and diffuse UV. This roof is lined in plywood to prevent heat radiating from the underside of the metal roofing. The heavy polished concrete floor shielded from the heat of the sun remains cool; this cool is radiated back to the occupants. The open sides allow breezes to further cool the space.

Key shade settings

Key shade settings are those that serve us, especially children and young adults, on a daily basis. In the domestic situation, an outdoor living space is a key shade setting. When considering the design of a new home or renovation, we should think of outdoor living spaces as an extension of the living area of the home so the family can move between them without having to use personal protection of sunscreen, hats or sunglasses. If the space is to be used for several hours over the middle of the day, then it is important to use a shading system that shields the direct sun and almost all the diffuse UVR (the view of the sky). Terraces or patios for eating breakfast and evening dinners can be open to low-angle sun and the open sky. At these times the UVI is low.

Key danger zones are in the open – on flat landscape, at the beach, on the water and in the mountains. Heavy personal protection is likely to be required at such places, and/or we should choose to experience them in the early morning and evening.

Making the change

People who are serious about becoming fully accustomed to the UVR levels can borrow or purchase a UV meter and test the UVR exposure at various times of day and year in everyday situations – on the terrace, at the beach or under a favourite shady tree (hand-held UV meters are available from http://www.solarmeter.com). This chapter has aimed to provide a general understanding but real-time measurements will consolidate it. People living in southern areas who are concerned about receiving enough UV exposure in the winter can calculate a sunbathing dose for vitamin D production.

Shade-seekers have an obligation to share their knowledge and behaviour with family and friends. In effect, we are developing long-term cultural traditions and customs to suit our relatively new homeland.

Further reading

Greenwood JS, Soulos GP, Thomas ND (1998) *Undercover: Guidelines for Shade Planning and Design*. Cancer Council NSW/NSW Health Department, Sydney.

Mackay C (2005) Living outside in the sun. *Idea*, 117–126. http://idea-edu.com/wp-content/uploads/2013/01/2005_IDEA_Journal.pdf.

Memmott P (2007) *Gunyah Goondie and Wurley: The Aboriginal Architecture of Australia*. UQP, Brisbane.

Plischke EA (1947) *Design and Living*. Department of Internal Affairs, Wellington.

Cancer Council websites provide information on shade design and resources relating to their region.

Chapter 7

The sun and eyes: sunlight-induced eye disease and its prevention

Minas Coroneo and Stephen Dain

Key messages

- For more than 150 years we have recognised that the harsh Australian sun has been causing eye problems.
- A wide range of eye health concerns has been linked to excessive direct and reflected UV radiation exposure and these often diminish sight.
- Good sun protection practice is important but special attention is required for good eye health for adults and children in our high-UV environment.
- Wrap-around sunglasses are important to block side light, which can be particularly damaging to the eye. Other high-quality protective eyewear is necessary in various circumstances, e.g. some occupational settings, and in high UV reflective environments, e.g. snow and water.
- The Australian standards in eye protection are very high and are a helpful guide when choosing good eye protection.

Evolution of the eye

Fans of Sir David Attenborough might imagine that, as fish evolved into amphibia and colonised the land, certain changes had to occur to the design of the eye. Since very little UV radiation (energetic and damaging wavelengths on the shorter side of violet) passes further than a metre or so through seawater, our eyes have benefited from the development of filters (to replace the protection of seawater) – a kind of inbuilt 'sunglass'.

Since vision is key to survival, effective filters meant reduced risk of disease and, therefore, better sight for longer. Thus, despite high levels of UV exposure, most Australians' eyes survive into old age, able to see but not always entirely unscathed by the sun's rays.

Only a partial solution to this problem evolved. In this chapter, we will outline the beneficial and harmful effects of sunlight and the best measures to protect the eyes from damage.

The basic problem is that, on the one hand, the eye requires light to see and to maintain eye and general health (circadian rhythms such as sleep cycles depend on blue-green light entering the eye). On the other hand, the eye can be damaged, particularly by both short (UV) and long (infrared) wavelengths.

As the human eye evolved, two features (perhaps 'design faults') have left the surface of the eye vulnerable to particular diseases.

Human eyes face forward. In order to improve side vision (creatures with side-pointing eyes already have good surround vision), the side of the human eye socket has been beautifully 'sculpted' away to improve our chance of seeing things to the sides (see Fig. 7.1). However, it increases exposure of the eye from the side, particularly to scattered UV radiation – this exposure is critical to development of certain diseases. The side exposure is more difficult to shield and attempts using wrap-around sunglasses have offered varying but often incomplete levels of protection.

The second problem relates to the fact that the 'whites' of our eyes are exposed so that an area known as the limbus (see Fig. 7.2) can be damaged by radiation exposure. The limbus is the meeting zone of the clear watchglass-like cornea and the opaque conjunctiva/sclera – more or less at the junction of the white with the coloured part of the eye. The coloured part of the eye is the iris, which is located inside the eye.

The limbus is home to a group of cells, known as stem cells, that replenish the surface of the eye. These cells divide and are eventually shed in the same way that we shed our skin. Their injury plays a critical role in the development of conditions known as pterygium (Fig. 7.3) and pinguecula (Fig. 7.6), both of which are caused by excessive exposure to the sun.

Pinguecula is a raised yellowish deposit on the inner aspect of the eye and may develop into a pterygium. Pterygium is a fleshy, often triangular-shaped overgrowth of altered conjunctiva, the

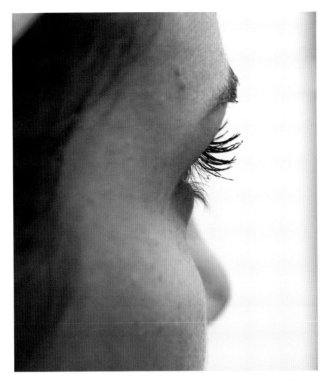

Fig. 7.1: Recession (cutting away) of the side aspect of the eye socket allows a wide field of view but increases the eye's exposure to UV radiation from the side.

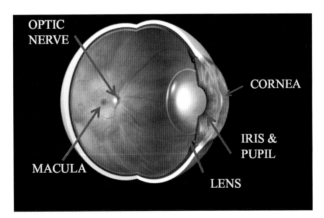

Fig. 7.2: Basic anatomy of the human eye. The eye is like a sophisticated and beautifully miniaturised camera. A double lens system, comprising the cornea and lens, focuses light onto the retina, a very sophisticated light-detecting 'chip'. The retina comprises the macula (a high-resolution zone for fine, detailed and colour vision) and the remainder that provides the lower-resolution but movement-sensitive side vision.

clear, blood vessel-containing membrane covering the white of the eye. It is sometimes referred to as 'surfer's eye'.

There is speculation as to the reason for this arrangement of cells in the eye. Most animal eyes have either eyelids or dark pigment hiding the white sclera and it can be hard to tell in which direction they are looking. This also protects the cells of the limbus. One theory is that the human eye evolved differently to play a role in communication – 'a nod is as good as a wink …'.

In recent times, partly fuelled by concerns over increased UV exposure as a result of the ozone hole, more attention has been placed on eye damage caused by the sun.

We have termed the conditions in which sunlight has been implicated (with varying degrees of certainty) in causing eye disease, the 'ophthalmohelioses' (from the Greek words ophthalmos = eye and helios = sun) (Table 7.1). This group of conditions has been of particularly great interest to Australian eye doctors, for reasons of history and climate.

Australia's first medical publication of 1840 stated:

> … in this climate the eye is more liable to be affected than in England. There is a Sun that for many months in the year shines with a power and a brilliancy, that 'at home' we are not cognizant of.

During her years in Australia, Ida Mann, first Professor of Ophthalmology at Oxford, recounted that it 'is the land of sin, sand, sorrow and sore eyes. It's the climate'.

Table 7.1: Sun-related eye conditions (ophthalmohelioses)

Eyelid	Wrinkles, baggy eyelids, sunburn, eyelid rotation out (ectropion), pre-cancerous changes, skin cancer, including melanoma malignancy
Eye surface	Pinguecula, pterygium, frosting of the cornea (climatic keratopathy [Labrador], snow blindness), pre-cancer and cancer, haze after laser surgery, onset of cold sore (herpes) virus infection, possible role in conical cornea (keratoconus)
Lens	Cataract, presbyopia (early need for reading glasses), glare associated with lens implanted after cataract surgery (dysphotopsia)
Retina	Eclipse blindness, melanoma inside the eye, macular degeneration, inflammation inside the eye (uveitis), possible role in glaucoma, floaters
Other	Short-sightedness from inadequate outdoor activity, shingles onset, migraine symptoms

An ophthalmologist, Dr Kerkenezov who practised in Lismore on the NSW north coast, was the first to observe (in 1956) that white people with pterygia (plural of pterygium) also suffered from skin cancer – an early clinical indication of the role of UV radiation in both conditions. Intriguingly, he also noted that pterygia developed about a decade before skin disease – the reason became apparent decades later.

Thus, an early link was made between UV exposure and both pterygium and skin cancer and, at that time, the link with melanoma of the skin was being proposed. It was also apparent that pterygium was most common between latitudes 40°N and 40°S and in island populations – a 'pterygium belt' straddles the equator, coinciding with the parts of the world exposed to the most intense UV radiation.

Yet much of the UV radiation that strikes the eye is reflected, indirect or diffuse radiation. This can cause sunburn even if a beach umbrella seems to be protecting you (see Chapters 4 and 6).

Studies by dermatologists in the 1960s showed that reflected radiation struck the eyes. It should come as no surprise that these sun-related eye conditions occur most commonly in places of high ground reflectance in people exposed under these conditions.

This may explain why there is a pterygium prevalence of 8.6% in Greenland at 61°N of the equator, compared with 7.3% in the Australian Blue Mountains. There is less than a third of direct UVB in Greenland compared with that found in the equatorial regions. Therefore, UV exposure may be similar if terrain reflectivity (like snow, which reflects UV radiation very effectively) is taken into account.

It has also been realised that, while we have been warned to avoid the midday sun when UV levels for skin peak, the situation of the eye differs. Eyes are located at a vantage point (so we can see better) and because of this, eye exposure to UV will vary greatly depending on time and season.

From spring to autumn, UV exposure of the eye is highest in the morning/evening, whereas in summer UV exposure is relatively small around noon, although the direct UV exposure is the strongest. In winter, eye UV exposure levels are maximal around noon.

Pterygium has been problematic since early settlement days, as Australia's first full-time ophthalmologist, Thomas Evans, described when reporting on a new operation in 1893 – a tradition continued by Arthur D'Ombrain in the 1940s. D'Ombrain noted:

> I have pinguecula (a fatty growth at the limbus) in both eyes; they formed in my
> twenty-second year when I possessed my first motor bicycle and before I learnt the

wisdom of wearing goggles; my late father, an ophthalmic surgeon, noticed the pinguecula and made me wear goggles.

This was perhaps early recognition of the importance of side light in ocular UV exposure and the fact that conventional spectacles offer inadequate protection.

Thus exposure from the side is likely to cause more damage than direct incident radiation and, clearly, this has implications for eye protection and sunglass design. A simple test of this idea is to go out on a bright day – if the terrain is particularly reflective, holding your hands up to the side of the face greatly reduces the brightness/glare and discomfort.

During the 1980s Fred Hollows described high pterygium prevalence rates in indigenous Australians and reasoned that the cause might be Aborigines 'spend all their waking hours outdoors caus[ing] them to be more exposed to solar radiation'. Yet when Aborigines were examined in South Australia in 1880s, pterygium was found to be uncommon.

It is possible that the earlier population had not been exposed to trachoma (an infection that can damage the limbus); perhaps a double insult to the limbus, first from infection then from UV exposure, may increase the risk of developing pterygium.

Another possible cause of the increase in pterygium rates is the westernisation of the diets of indigenous Australians, with a resultant reduction in 'internal' protection from UV radiation: diet plays a role in the antioxidant levels in our skin and may help protect against sun damage.

Peripheral light focusing and the development of pterygium

During the 1980s, we noticed that light incident from the side was focused by the front of the eye to areas at the limbus and in the lens of the eye on the other side (closest to the nose).

Thus the optics of the eye work 'side-on' as well as 'front-on'. In the front-on mode, light is focused onto the retina (just as a camera lens focuses light onto a chip or film in a camera). We realised that these foci (10–20 times more intense than normal incident light) coincided with the usual sites of pterygium (Fig. 7.3) and a particular type of cataract. A cataract is an opacity of the lens of the eye; a healthy lens is normally transparent (Fig. 7.4).

Both these conditions affect only a sector of the eye on the side closest to the nose. Until this discovery, there had not been a plausible explanation for this location. In both cases, there is focal

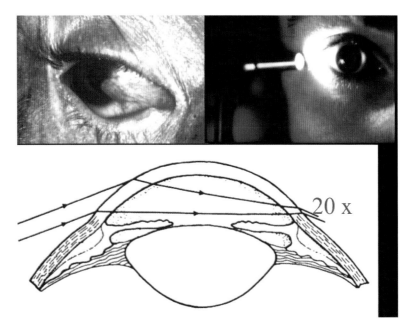

Fig. 7.3: (Top left) A typical pterygium, a fleshy inflamed mass invading the nasal side of the cornea. (Top right) Light from a torch aimed at the outer side of the cornea, being focused by the front of the eye to the other side of the cornea, resulting in a bright spot at the limbus, coincident with the usual location of pterygium. (Bottom) The light pathways. The intensity of the light at this spot is 20× the intensity of the light striking the other side of the eye.

damage to the stem cells that renew these areas of tissue. These focusing effects were termed the 'Coroneo effect' by Fred Hollows.

Both pterygium and cataract reduce vision. Pterygium can grow across the line of sight and/or distort the cornea and cataract blocks light from reaching the retina directly. It may also be associated with glare, as it causes light to scatter. Both conditions are common and ultimately may require surgery.

Pterygium can cause quite marked redness of the eyes as sunlight induces inflammation of the tissue exposed ('eye sunburn'). This can also result in symptoms of dryness of the eye. Many patients with pterygium develop symptoms in smoky, dusty environments and are often concerned about the cosmetic appearance of their red, watery eyes.

Because the eye provides the only focusing system in the body (allowing 10–20× intensification of light), these eye conditions would be expected to occur before skin damage, thus an explanation for Dr Kerkenezov's findings from the 1950s. Also, if the ozone hole were exposing

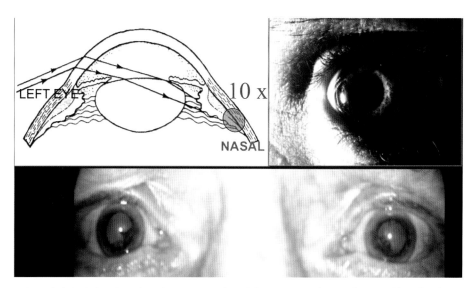

Fig. 7.4: (Top right) Light aimed at the outer side of the cornea, being focused by the front of the eye to the other side of the lens (within the eye), resulting in a bright red spot appearing in the sclera (white of the eye), coincident with the usual early location of cataract. (Top left) The light pathways. The intensification of the light is 10× (perhaps accounting for the fact that cataract onset occurs later in life than pterygium – focusing effect responsible is 20×). The light spot is red, as the light has to pass through a layer of blood vessels before it reaches the surface of the eye. (Bottom) Opaque areas in the inner part of the 'red reflex' of the eye (within the pupil), representing early cataract, typically located in the area of the lens closest to the nose.

us to more UV radiation, we would expect an increase in these eye conditions before a rise in skin cancer prevalence.

We can detect early damage to the surface of the eye (at the limbus) in children as young as nine (Fig. 7.5), using special photographic techniques. By age 15, ~80% of children in one Sydney area showed these changes. Why don't all these children develop pterygium? The answer may lie in the fact that there are natural repair mechanisms that may help heal the body during times of low UV exposure. There may also be genetic susceptibility – pterygium tends to run in families. Other factors such as diet may play a role.

Other conditions

Table 7.1 listed a range of eye conditions for which UV exposure may be at least partly responsible. For the eyelids, these range from the relatively trivial such as wrinkles and baggy

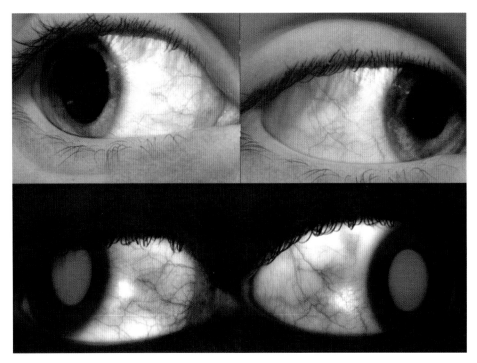

Fig. 7.5: (Top) Normal-looking eyes in a nine-year-old patient. (Bottom) When photos are taken in UV light, areas on the inner part of the eye light up. These areas are thought to represent early damage caused by sun exposure. In time, further damage in these locations may result in formation of a pinguecula (Fig. 7.6) that may go on to develop into pterygium.

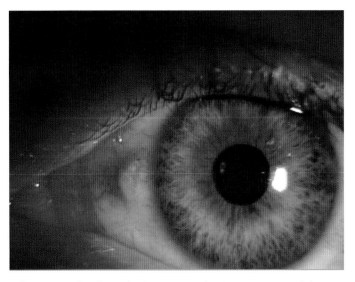

Fig. 7.6: A pinguecula, a raised yellowish deposit on the inner aspect of the eye, adjacent to the cornea. A pinguecula may be a precursor of pterygium.

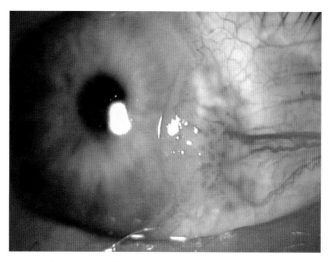

Fig. 7.7: Cancerous area at the inner limbus – while the location is the same as for pterygium or pinguecula, it can typically occur anywhere near the limbus. The appearance is entirely different from that of a pterygium.

eyelids (cosmetic surgery is often performed for these conditions), to various types of skin cancer. Eyelid skin cancer, although usually treatable, may create serious problems for the surface of the eye even after eyelid reconstruction. Furthermore, the cancer may grow into the eye socket and become incurable. It may result in loss of the eye and, occasionally, loss of life.

The surface of the eye may be affected by pterygium, as noted, and by a pre-pterygium fatty change (pinguecula). This is mostly of cosmetic concern but can grow into a pterygium.

Just like the skin, the surface of the eye may develop forms of cancer (Fig. 7.7) – typically adjacent to the limbus. A small percentage of pterygium cases harbour cancerous or pre-cancerous cells. Fortunately, these spots respond very well to medical treatment and don't usually need surgery. Melanoma of the surface of the eye is very uncommon.

Skiers (who require goggles rather than sunglasses for adequate protection) or welders who do not wear face shields can develop extremely painful 'snow blindness', in which the surface layer of the eye is damaged by UV radiation, exposing nerve endings. This usually heals without permanent damage.

Long-term exposure, e.g. in places like Labrador in northern Canada, may cause a more permanent frosting of the cornea. This is likely due to the high levels of UV reflectance off the snow which is present much of the year. Similarly, corneal haze may occur in patients who have had laser surgery (e.g. for short-sightedness) and, although this usually settles with treatment, permanent changes may occur.

UV exposure may play a role in activation of a herpes virus infection of the eye surface.

Damage to the lens may manifest as cataract, in which the lens becomes opaque. This occurs particularly in the area adjacent to the nose. Not all cataracts are due to sun exposure, the commonest associations are with old age and smoking. Cataract may also be associated with taking certain drugs such as steroids and in medical conditions such as diabetes.

Although cataract surgery is perhaps the most successful of any procedure ever developed for replacing a body part, surgery is usually only performed when symptoms warrant intervention.

Another condition affecting the lens is presbyopia (age-related reduction in near/reading vision). This occurs as a consequence of lens hardening/stiffening, along with a possible reduction in the power of the muscle that surrounds the lens. This process may particularly accelerate in hot sunny climates. Whereas most people with normal sight require reading glasses in their 40s, this may occur earlier in such locations. It is probably the hotness of the climate rather than the sunniness that causes this effect.

The role of sunlight in causing damage to the front of the eye is now well established, but there is less evidence that sun damages the back/inner eye. The most obvious form of damage results from staring directly at the sun – a condition known as eclipse blindness. Despite warnings not to gaze at the sun during eclipses, the behaviour remains surprisingly common. While some recovery of vision can occur, permanent damage to the macula (the part of the retina that is used for fine detailed vision; see Fig. 7.8) is usual. It is essentially untreatable.

Another macular condition, age-related macular degeneration, is the commonest cause of legal blindness in most western societies.

It is uncertain why macular degeneration occurs. Several factors play a role, including age, nutrition and smoking. The role of sunlight remains controversial but possible. Much of the evidence is indirect – a recent study of French alpine mountain guides showed that they had more damage to the front of the eye as well as macular degenerative changes when compared with a control population living in the adjacent valleys. Sunlight was implicated in causing both types of disease.

Other indirect evidence comes from the fact that many elderly patients take medications for their general health (e.g. for blood pressure control), some of which may increase susceptibility to light damage (photosensitisation), hence contributing to macular damage.

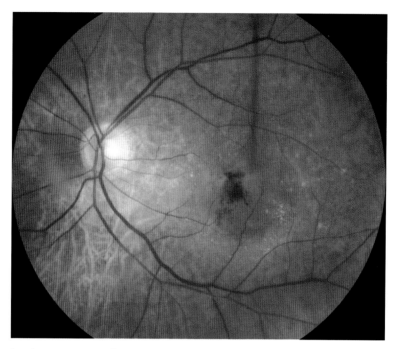

Fig. 7.8: Macular degeneration. The macula is to the right of the optic nerve and is looking at the end of a target (straight line from above). Surrounding the fixating point are degenerative areas of yellowish deposit (typical of the 'dry' or slow form of this disease). At the end of the pointer is a small haemorrhage, seen in the 'wet', a rapidly progressing form of the disease.

While melanoma of the inner eye is uncommon, there is some evidence that sunlight exposure may play a role.

Floaters (spots, specks or web-like structures that float around inside the eye) are a common condition due, it is thought, to a degeneration of the vitreous. Vitreous is the clear gel that occupies the space between the retina and the lens inside the eye. This degeneration may be hastened by UV exposure.

Uveitis is an inflammation that occurs in the middle layer of the wall of the eye (and includes the iris). It may be more common in the summer months and this may mean that sunlight plays a contributing role in some cases.

Glaucoma is a condition in which (usually) elevated eye pressure causes damage to the nerves inside the eye. It is a common problem. In most cases sunlight is unlikely to play a major role but there is indirect evidence that light entering the eye may cause some damage to the valve structure that controls eye pressure, so a possible role has not been excluded.

Lack of sunlight, or at least lack of time spent outdoors, has been implicated as a contributing factor to the development of short-sightedness (myopia).

This abbreviated list of conditions (Table 7.1, p. 116) summarises the range of diseases in which sunlight damage is implicated, often with a consequential reduction of vision.

The conditions of pterygium and cataract, and their observed location, provide clues to how this damage occurs. This has clear implications for the type of protection that may help to prevent these diseases.

Protecting the eye against UV radiation

As discussed, the effects of UV on the eye are both short-term and long-term and specific to each structure of the eye. The ways of preventing or reducing these effects are also specific to the structures.

Avoid the risk

The first protection strategy is avoidance. That is, we minimise or eliminate our exposure to the risk. We need to avoid the part of the day with the highest UV dose (generally, but not always, around the middle of the day – for longer periods during summer and shorter periods in winter, or using the UV Index when the UVI is 3 or higher).

General measures

To a certain extent UV exposure can be reduced by the use of shade structures. The use of a broad-brimmed hat will approximately halve the dose to the eyes.

In general, painted structures are poor reflectors of UV except when the reflection is of a low sun on a gloss or UV-reflecting paint. Metal surfaces such as galvanised iron are effective UV reflectors; building designers need to pay attention to where the sun will be reflected.

Protection against short-term effects of excessive UV

In the case of short-term consequences (i.e. within a day) there are two main effects. The first occurs when the front of the eye is exposed, resulting in painful snow blindness. It is caused by exposure to highly reflective snow or in the work environment with exposure to welding. The second is eclipse blindness, caused by exposure of the retina when viewing the sun directly.

Snow blindness

As discussed, the effects on the front of the eye (sometimes referred to as snow blindness) are caused by UV on the cornea and conjunctiva, so both structures need protecting. Contact lenses (except the very rare ones that cover the whole of the front of the eye) will not protect the conjunctiva. The conjunctiva is more sensitive to damage than the cornea, so contact lens wearers still need additional protection such as sunglasses or, at work, tinted eye protectors.

Selection of personal eye protection against UV in the natural environment will be discussed later since protection against the longer-term effects of UV has the same principles. Personal eye protection from artificial sources of UV using welding filters, UV filters and protective eye wear for solaria will also be discussed later.

Eclipse blindness

Viewing eclipses unprotected is a significant cause of damage to the retina. It should be emphasised that viewing the sun unprotected is always a significant risk whether or not a solar eclipse is occurring. Viewing during the period of totality (total coverage of the sun by the moon) must only be done with appropriate guidance. There is no Australian standard for eclipse viewing filters, so not all eclipse viewing glasses sold in Australia will be helpful in reducing harm linked with viewing an eclipse. During recent eclipses in Australia, eclipse viewing glasses that complied with European standard EN 1836 were available. Eclipse glasses meeting that standard provide adequate protection. If you want to view an eclipse, do so only through viewing glasses that meet the requirements of EN 1836.

A welding filter of shade 12 or darker also provides appropriate protection when viewing an eclipse.

Glare

Glare is a consequence of visible light, rather than UV, landing on the eye. Glare comes in two forms – discomfort glare and disability glare.

Discomfort glare is, as the name suggests, the discomfort or even pain that we experience as a result of a very bright light. Preventing this discomfort is often the main motivation for people to wear sunglasses.

Disability glare reduces vision and occurs when light is scattered in the eye by diseases such as cataract or simply by dirty or scratched spectacle lenses. The scattered light is spread over the retina and dilutes the contrast of the image. This effect is not lessened by wearing sunglasses since they will reduce the scattered light and the light of the image itself in the same proportion.

Disability glare is also caused by reflection from a surface such as water or the glossy page of a magazine. Objects in the water or images on the page are obscured by the reflection. Polarising lenses (discussed later) are a useful option in this case.

Selecting personal protection

Sunglasses and fashion spectacles

By law, all sunglasses and fashion spectacles sold in Australia must comply with the Consumer Product Safety Standard. This incorporates most of AS/NZS 1067. The provisions include UV protection. Australia is unique in the world in having a legally imposed sunglass standard that is implemented by the Australian Competition and Consumer Commission (ACCC) and the state Offices of Fair Trading (the title varies between states).

Sunglasses may be a uniform tint or a gradient tint. They may be polarising (dealing especially with glare reflected from horizontal surfaces) and/or photochromic (they go darker when exposed to sunlight). Every sunglass is required to carry information, usually on a swing tag. Looking for and understanding this information is key to choosing successful UV and sunglare protection. Sunglasses and fashion spectacles without such information fail the requirements of the standard and should not be on the market.

The information will have a category number (that indicates the level of protection) and a brief description to guide your selection (see Table 7.2).

Photochromic lenses change their visible tint according to the level of sunlight in the environment where they are worn. They must be labelled as 'photochromic' and carry two category numbers corresponding to the inactivated and activated states. Photochromic lenses may be useful when going from dark to light repeatedly, but they lighten relatively slowly. In a car, the protection of the roof and the windscreen (which itself has a high level of UV absorption) remove the radiation that makes the lens go dark. The lenses are also less effective in high temperatures.

Sunglasses and fashion spectacles that do not meet certain colour requirements are required to carry the warning MUST NOT BE USED WHEN DRIVING and carry the symbol shown in Table 7.2.

Table 7.2: Key information in choosing sunglasses

Lens category	Description required on label	Other information required	Comments
0	Fashion spectacles – not sunglasses Very low sun glare protection Some UV protection	None	These are untinted or very pale tints. They are not designed for sun glare protection but are required to give some UV protection. They are worn mostly for cosmetic reasons or wind protection
1	Fashion spectacles – not sunglasses Limited sun glare protection Some UV protection	NOT SUITABLE FOR DRIVING AT NIGHT	These are pale tints. They are of little use for sun glare protection but are required to give some UV protection. Tints of any kind should not be worn driving at night
2	Sunglasses Medium sun glare protection Good UV protection	None	These are typical sunglasses providing appropriate levels of sun glare and UV protection. Category 3 is darker than category 2
3	Sunglasses High sun glare protection Good UV protection		
4	Sunglasses – special purpose Very high sun glare protection Good UV protection	MUST NOT BE USED WHEN DRIVING and carry the symbol	These are very dark sunglasses for very bright situations. They are too dark for driving

Finally, sunglasses and fashion spectacles must carry the name and address of an Australian company.

Sunglasses must meet optical quality and robustness requirements but it is important to realise that they do not necessarily meet the higher impact requirements of occupational eye protection – sunglasses and fashion spectacles are not appropriate eye protection in the workplace. Eye protectors that comply with AS/NZS 1337.1 and are sun glare protectors (see 'Occupational eye protection', p. 131) are better options at work.

Sunglasses may carry claims such as '100% UV protection'. The standard provides methods and criteria by which such claims may be assessed. However, there is no agreed criterion or test for the common claim of 'UV400'. It has no clear meaning.

The ACCC has recalled some sunglasses and eye protectors because they did not meet the standard: check at http://www.recalls.gov.au/content/index.phtml/itemId/952797 or add the words 'recall, government and sunglasses' into a search engine.

The standard ensures that the lenses are appropriate and specifies minimum size requirements, but some simple guidelines can also be applied.

Visible light and UV can reach the eye from around the frame and lenses. The best protection comes from a larger frame that fits closely to the face and provides protection from the side in the form of a wrap-around design, side shields or broad sides.

Many sunglasses wrap around at the sides or have windows in the side arms, offering some protection against scattered or reflected side radiation. However, if the eye can be seen when the wearer has sunglasses on, it is likely that UV radiation can reach the eye around the edge of the sunglasses, allowing 'light focusing' to cause damage (Fig. 7.9). Simply wearing wrap-around sunglasses without checking this point may give a false sense of security.

Polarising lenses are helpful when there is reflected glare, especially from water or shiny bitumen roads. They may, however, cause problems with the visibility of some LCD displays in cars or digital watches.

Contact lenses

Not all contact lenses are UV-absorbing; those that are, are usually specifically labelled. It is generally a good idea for wearers to choose contact lenses that offer good UV protection.

Rigid contact lenses are generally smaller and cover only the centre of the cornea. The better options are UV-absorbing soft contact lenses that cover the cornea, some of the conjunctiva and, most importantly, the all-important limbus at the edge of the cornea.

As not all contact lenses are effective in protecting against pterygium, where practicable wearers should also use good-quality sunglasses for prolonged periods outdoors. This is particularly important around water environments, where the low sun is reflected from the water to the eye, and around sand, light-coloured soils and snow that have a high UV reflection.

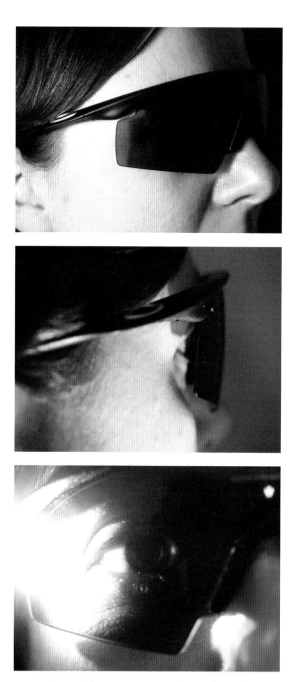

Fig. 7.9: Inadequate eye protection with a wrap-around sunglass design. (Top) A commonly available sunglass design. (Middle) Eye exposure evident by viewing from the side. If the eye can be seen, UV rays of light can reach it. (Bottom) Light focusing at the limbus caused by a side light located beyond the edge of the sunglass frame.

Since protection against glare requires a significant reduction of visible light, tinted contact lenses, being inconvenient to remove and replace when moving to and from sunlight, are not a realistic option.

Ski goggles

The UV requirements of ski goggle standards are more stringent than of sunglass standards. The category numbers (which are based on the amount of visible light transmitted) are the same as for sunglasses and fashion spectacles. There is a specific warning not to use ski goggles when driving.

Australia and New Zealand have no standard for ski goggles. Buyers should look for claims of compliance with the European standard EN 174 or the US ASTM F659. The ISO is working on ISO 18527–1 and this will probably be used to create an Australian/New Zealand standard in the foreseeable future.

Occupational eye protection

These days, eye protectors and sunglasses may be indistinguishable. Eye protectors that are also sun glare protectors have to meet much the same UV and visible light requirements as sunglasses and fashion spectacles. But the impact protection requirements are greater for occupation eye protection. There are two grades of impact protection applicable to occupational eye protection. Low impact is required of every eye protector; there may be the letter 'S' on the lens. Medium impact is an optional grade; such eye protectors may be identified via an 'I' or 'F' on the lens.

Colouration requirements for eye protectors are also more stringent. As a consequence, tinted eye protectors are completely adequate as sunglasses but sunglasses are not necessarily adequate as occupational eye protectors. The relevant standard is AS/NZS 1337.1.

Untinted eye protectors do not have to meet any UV requirements. They may be marked 'O' for 'Outdoor use' to indicate that they include sufficient UV protection. They will identify the manufacturer on the lenses and frame.

Guidance on the selection of appropriate eye protection is given in the standard AS/NZS 1336.

Prescription spectacles and sunglasses

Generally prescription lenses, even untinted (with the exception of glass, which is rarely used these days) have good UV absorption built in. The visible light categories are the same as for sunglasses and fashion spectacles, but the UV performance may be different. There is no mandatory standard for prescription spectacles or sunglasses. Expect the supplier of prescription lenses to confirm that the lenses comply with the non-mandatory AS/NZS ISO 8980.3.

Prescription eye protection

For UV protection and visible transmission, including categories, the requirements are exactly the same as for non-prescription eye protectors. The impact categories and lens markings requirements are the same except that they will also carry the letter 'R' to indicate that they are eye protectors as well as prescription lenses. AS/NZS 1337.6 applies to prescription eye protection.

Eye protection in solaria

Commercial solaria are banned from the end of 2014 in Australia (see Ch. 3). However, at the time of writing they remain legal in New Zealand and a small number of people may have a solarium in their home. AS/NZS 2635 has requirements for eye protectors used in solaria but there are no requirements for labelling, so it is unclear how the user can decide if the supplied eye protectors comply. The requirements are written differently and, in some respects, are more stringent than for sunglasses. Sunglasses may not provide adequate eye protection. The standard places the onus of compliance on the solarium operator.

Sunglasses and children

Children are particularly sensitive to UV radiation skin and eye damage, so it is important to protect children's eyes. Exposure of very young children to UV radiation should be limited. They should wear a sun-smart hat to provide some protection to the eyes.

Once children are old enough to manage wearing sunglasses, they should be encouraged to do so when exposed to UV radiation. These glasses should meet the recommendations above. Sunglasses labelled as toys are not covered by the standard and therefore should not be used to provide sun protection.

Issues with sunglasses

While eye protection against UV radiation is a good idea (and sunglasses offer much greater eye protection than a hat), there have been recent concerns raised about their use by those who care for patients who have developed melanoma of the skin.

Some are concerned that the act of putting on sunglasses reduces visible light glare and turns off the skin exposure warning-system of excessive brightness. This may result in the wearer spending more time in the sun, which increases skin UV exposure. If the side protection is inadequate, there may be increased exposure of the eye as the normal reflex of squinting (i.e. half-closing the eyes in bright environments) is reduced.

There is also some evidence that pupil size increases in sunglass wearers, which may result in increased amounts of UV entering the eye. Particularly dark tints reduce our ability to see. Frames with wide side arms will reduce side vision.

Many beachgoers do not wear sunglasses because of inconvenience and the risk of dirt, damage and theft, especially with expensive sunglasses. There is great scope to develop better eye protection for people engaged in popular outdoor activities in climates and environments such as in Australia.

The relevance of diet

Early studies linked certain dietary deficiencies, including choline deficiency, with development of pterygium. Because inflammation is associated with pterygium growth and symptoms, medical treatments that safely suppress inflammation may stabilise this condition. The anti-inflammatory attributes of Mediterranean and traditional diets, which are generally high in plant-based foods in which choline has been identified, may play a role in protecting against the severity or progression of pterygium.

Sunlight-induced processes, such as oxidative stress in the eye, could trigger inflammation that choline-deficient people are less able to counter.

It has been suggested that the low rates of melanoma found in Mediterranean countries may be partly due to the protective effect of the Mediterranean diet. After carefully controlling for several sun exposure and pigmentary characteristics, researchers have established that there is a protective effect given by the weekly consumption of fish and shellfish, the daily drinking of tea and a high consumption of vegetables, in particular cabbages and other leafy vegetables and fruits (especially citrus fruits).

There is strong circumstantial evidence that omega-3 fatty acids are protective against the development of the non-melanoma skin cancers, such as basal cell and squamous cell carcinomas, which can affect both the eyelids and ocular surface.

There is some evidence that the anti-oxidant properties of vitamins C and E may protect against the development and progression of cataract. Eating five or more servings of well-chosen fruits and vegetables each day, as recommended by many authorities, should provide more than 100 mg vitamin C and 5–6 mg of carotenoids, including lutein and zeaxanthin. Eating two servings of nuts and seeds will provide 8–14 mg vitamin E.

Similar advice applies to age-related macular degeneration (ARMD). The Macular Disease Foundation recommends a healthy, well-balanced diet with dark green leafy vegetables and fresh fruit daily and fish two to three times a week. We should choose low glycemic index (low GI) carbohydrates instead of high GI, eat a handful of nuts a week and limit our intake of fats and oils.

The link between smoking and ARMD is well established, as it is with cataracts – the quit-smoking message is important for eye health.

Diet may provide internal protection against UV damage and is a strong additional measure to the external protective measures described above. Healthy lifestyle choices in relation to diet, weight and exercise may result in improved eye health.

Conclusion

In recent years there has been a better understanding of the effects of UV on eye health. Some of this information is not obvious and some is even counter-intuitive. In this chapter we have summarised research findings and made recommendations in relation to protective measures.

Research results have affected sunglass standards and may result in improved sunglass and contact lens designs in the near future. The emerging role of diet in mitigating sun damage will be of interest in the years to come and will link the sun-protection message with public health messages on the benefit of good diet to general health.

Improved early detection methods for sun damage to the eye may provide opportunities to 'get in early' and stop disease progression before there is a significant effect on sight.

Further reading

Attenborough D (2009) *Charles Darwin and the Tree of Life*. DVD, BBC Home Entertainment.

Coroneo MT (2011) Ultraviolet radiation and the anterior eye. *Eye and Contact Lens* **37**, 214–224. doi:10.1097/ICL.0b013e318223394e.

Coroneo MT, Coroneo H (2010) *Feast Your Eyes: The Eye Health Cookbook*. Seaview Press, Adelaide.

Dain SJ (2003) Sunglasses and sunglass standards. *Clinical and Experimental Optometry* **86**, 77–90. doi:10.1111/j.1444-0938.2003.tb03066.x.

Chapter 8

Vitamin D, health and the sun: finding the right balance

Rachel Neale and Robyn Lucas

Key messages

- Vitamin D plays a key role in maintaining the right levels of calcium in the blood, which is important for good bone health.
- Most Australians get their vitamin D through exposure of the skin to the sun.
- There is ongoing research into whether vitamin D is important for other conditions. There is much scientific debate on other health issues and their relationship to vitamin D.
- Vitamin D levels below 30 nmol/L are considered deficient and need to be addressed by a doctor.
- Levels above 100 nmol/L may be excessive and equally may need medical attention.
- Modest amounts of sun exposure are necessary to obtain sufficient vitamin D. Many factors influence exactly how much sun is needed.
- It is possible to maintain adequate vitamin D production without substantially increasing skin cancer risk.
- Being sun-smart is not about hiding in the cupboard under the stairs all the time, but about getting a modest amount of sun without overexposure to the extreme levels of UV radiation common in Australia and New Zealand through our summer period.

Introduction

Vitamin D, sometimes known as the sunshine vitamin because it is produced in the skin after sun exposure, was discovered ~100 years ago. We've known for many decades that it plays a major role in ensuring strong and healthy bones in children and adults. Due to scientific research in the last two decades, it is now thought to have far wider-ranging health benefits. In this chapter we will consider some of these and highlight some of the challenges in deciding how much vitamin D we need and the best way to achieve an ideal level.

The discovery of vitamin D

Vitamin D was discovered by scientists as they tried to find a way to prevent or cure rickets, a disease that causes deformed bones in children (Fig. 8.1). Rickets has afflicted children for a very long time, with descriptions of deformed bones appearing as early as the first century. However, it wasn't until the middle of the 17th century that the first scientific description of rickets was published. With increasing industrialisation in Europe through the 18th century, people moved

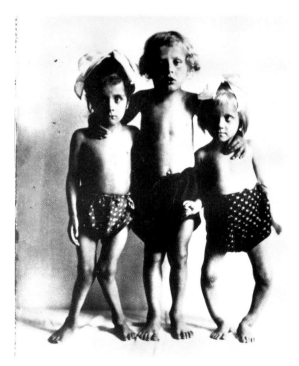

Fig. 8.1: Three children with rickets, c.1920–30. Wellcome Library, London.

from country areas to large polluted cities. They swapped their rural lifestyles for long hours indoors, for example in factories. Rickets then became common.

In the mid 1800s, cod liver oil was given as a tonic to prevent rickets, and the disease was noted to be less common in sunnier locations. Some experiments in the early 1900s confirmed the beneficial effects of cod liver oil.

The active ingredient was identified and, because it was the fourth vitamin discovered, it was called vitamin D. A short time later, scientists observed that exposing the skin to UV radiation caused a substance equivalent to vitamin D to be produced. In the century since these seminal discoveries, a vast body of research has been carried out to understand how vitamin D is processed in the body, how it affects the functions of cells and, most importantly, how it influences human health.

Vitamin D metabolism

Vitamin D is different from most other vitamins because our bodies can make it, although we can also obtain it from foods or supplements. Vitamin D comes in two forms, vitamin D3 (also called cholecalciferol) and vitamin D2 (also called ergocalciferol). When skin is exposed to UV radiation (present in sunlight) vitamin D3 is produced. Only a small number of foods contain vitamin D3. The best sources are oily fish such as salmon and mackerel, but milk and egg yolks also contain a small amount of vitamin D3. Vitamin D2 is found in plants, mainly mushrooms, that have been exposed to UV radiation.

Irrespective of whether vitamin D is made in the skin or ingested, or whether we obtain it as vitamin D3 or vitamin D2, it must undergo some processing in the body before it is active (Fig. 8.2). It is transported in the bloodstream to the liver where it is converted to 25 hydroxy vitamin D (25D). This molecule circulates in the blood and can be converted in the kidneys to the biologically active form of vitamin D, 1,25 dihydroxy vitamin D (1,25D). For a long time it was thought that this second step had to occur in the kidneys, but we now know that many different types of cells have the chemicals needed to convert 25D to 1,25D.

How do we measure vitamin D?

The concentration in blood of the intermediate form, 25D, is thought to provide the best measure of both circulating and stored (in fat tissue) vitamin D. The concentration is usually reported in

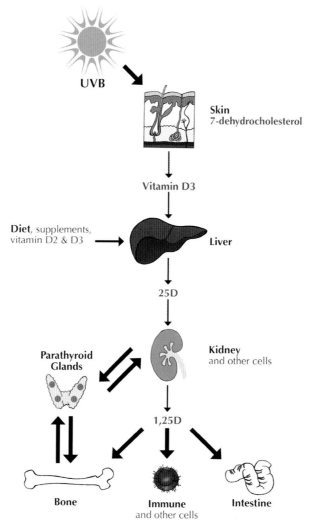

Fig. 8.2: The pathway from UVB exposure from the sun to the creation of 1,25D, the biologically important component of vitamin D that benefits our health.

Australia in nanomoles per litre (nmol/L). In the USA, nanograms per millilitre (ng/mL) is used. To convert from ng/mL to nmol/L, multiply by 2.5:

$$20 \text{ ng/mL} = 20 \times 2.5 = 50 \text{ nmol/L}$$

There are many different methods for measuring the concentration of 25D. Unfortunately, 25D is quite a difficult chemical to measure and the result can vary according to the type of method used. Different laboratories using the same method can get different results, and even within one laboratory the results of the test can vary over time due to the different batches of reagents used. There are more accurate methods but they are not in common use because they are labour-intensive and expensive.

Blood levels of 25D reflect vitamin D intake and sun exposure over the previous six to eight weeks.

Recently an international Vitamin D Standardisation Program has been developed by the leading national health authorities in the USA. Thus, over the next few years we should expect major improvements in the accuracy of vitamin D testing in Australia and elsewhere. In the meantime, the lack of accuracy in vitamin D measurement is of major concern because public health and clinical decisions are being based on tests that do not necessarily reflect the person's true vitamin D status.

What does vitamin D do in our bodies?

The primary function of the active form of vitamin D (1,25D) is to maintain the right levels of calcium in the blood to allow cells to function normally. Maintaining stable calcium levels in the blood is extremely important for the body's normal functioning and calcium levels are constantly monitored (by sensors in the parathyroid gland that sits within the thyroid gland in the neck). When calcium levels drop, parathyroid hormone is released and this causes the kidneys to increase the conversion of 25D to 1,25D. The active 1,25D acts on the gut so that it increases the uptake of calcium in food or supplements and on the kidneys to minimise the loss of calcium in the urine. When there is not enough calcium in the diet to get calcium levels back to normal, 1,25D causes specialised bone cells (osteoclasts) to mature. These can break down bone to release the calcium stored there.

We know that having enough vitamin D is important to keeping our bones in good condition. For a long time this seemed to be its only role. In the last 10–15 years, however, vitamin D deficiency has been linked to an increased risk of many diseases such as cancers, heart disease, immune and mental health disorders, and others. We briefly review the evidence for some of these below.

Vitamin D and bone health

Bones are remodelled constantly throughout our lives, so much so that most of the adult skeleton is replaced every 10 years. It is very important that we have enough calcium to allow new bone to

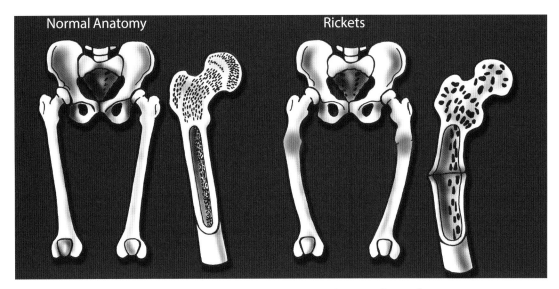

Fig. 8.3: Healthy bones compared to bones affected by rickets. Redrawn from http://centerforchildren.med.nyu.edu/rickets.

be formed and for that bone to be strong. Not having enough vitamin D, either through lack of sun exposure or not having enough in the diet or as a supplement, can lead to vitamin D deficiency. This may result in very little calcium being absorbed in the gut and not having enough calcium available to be incorporated in newly forming bone (Fig. 8.3). The result is soft bones that bend easily. In children this causes rickets, with its typical appearance of knock-knees or bandy legs. In adults the same condition is called osteomalacia. It causes pain in the bones, weak muscles and tiredness and the bones may fracture very easily.

If low calcium levels in the blood cannot be remedied by increasing the uptake of calcium (from food or supplements) in the gut (either because of vitamin D deficiency or there is not enough calcium in the diet) and minimising the calcium lost in the urine, calcium can be drawn out of the bones. That is, calcium levels in the blood will be maintained at the expense of bone strength. If this goes on for some time it results in osteomalacia, or rickets of adulthood.

Vitamin D and cancer

Of course, this book is largely about a specific type of cancer – skin cancer. Generally, and as described in Chapter 1, cancer is caused when damage to the DNA of a cell causes it to lose its ability to control its own growth. This cell can divide uncontrollably, giving rise to other (daughter) cells which are similarly unregulated. The result is often the development of an abnormal growth somewhere in the body. The other hallmark of most cancers is their ability to spread elsewhere in the body (metastasise) and form a new growth in a distant organ.

Studies in cells and laboratory animals indicate that vitamin D may have anti-cancer properties. For example, exposing a cell with DNA damage to vitamin D can help it to die before it is able to produce daughter cells. Vitamin D might also be able to stop the formation of blood vessels that support growth of the tumour. However, experiments in cells or mice don't necessarily tell us what the situation will be in humans.

In the past decade there have been many studies that have investigated whether D deficiency is associated with the risk of cancer. Most have been prospective cohort studies, in which a large number of people are recruited, answer a survey and donate a blood sample. They are then followed forward in time ('prospectively') to see if they do or don't get cancer. The 25D level in the baseline blood sample of those who get cancer is then compared with the level in the blood of those who don't.

The most consistent evidence for an association between vitamin D and cancer is for cancer of the colon (large bowel) where most studies show that people who had higher 25D levels were at lower risk of developing colon cancer. For other cancers the evidence is inconsistent. For some, such as pancreatic cancer, some studies (although not all) have shown that people with high levels of 25D are actually at increased risk of cancer.

The big problem with cohort studies is that there are many factors apart from vitamin D that influence risk of disease, and some of these also affect 25D levels. For example, we know that people who are overweight or obese are at greater risk of developing colon cancer. These people also have lower levels of vitamin D. So is it the low vitamin D that increases the risk of colon cancer or is low vitamin D simply a marker of being unhealthy?

One way to overcome this problem is to use a different type of study where the researcher randomly (by chance) assigns some study participants to receive a vitamin D supplement and some to receive a placebo (non-active) tablet. This should mean similar numbers of overweight or generally less healthy people in both groups. By comparing the two 'treatment' groups, we can see if there is a difference in how many people develop the disease.

Few of these randomised trials have been large enough to assess the effect of vitamin D supplementation on cancer risk. One, the Women's Health Initiative trial in the USA, was big enough (it involved over 36 000 post-menopausal women) and it did not find that vitamin D supplementation reduced risk of cancer. However, it has been argued that the dose of vitamin D used was too low and that many people didn't take their assigned tablets. These possible explanations suggest that the findings of this trial might be unreliable. Several large trials have now been launched around the world, including one in Australia, that will help to answer the question about whether taking a vitamin D supplement can reduce the risk of cancer.

Vitamin D and the immune system

The human immune system is really two systems, which are separate but have lots of communication between them. The 'innate' immune system is similar to that found in all animals and has been around a long time, in evolutionary terms. It forms a first line of defence against threats such as infection by viruses or bacteria (pathogens) and is made up of specific immune cells and chemicals that engulf and destroy microbes. The innate immune response is fast, non-specific (treats all pathogens or threats the same) and 'all-or-none'.

Mammals, including humans, have also developed an 'adaptive' immune system, consisting of antibodies and cells that 'learn' with each successive contact with a particular pathogen. When we first encounter a pathogen the adaptive immune response – mainly seen as the development of antibodies – takes days to weeks to develop. The next time we are exposed to that pathogen there is a specific, targeted, rapid and effective immune response. This is the basis of vaccination – some part of the pathogen, or sometimes a killed version of the pathogen, is presented to the immune system. Antibodies are produced that will recognise the real pathogen if it tries to infect, and these then rapidly and effectively destroy that pathogen.

The active form of vitamin D has a wide variety of effects on the immune system. In general, it helps the innate immune system to work better, by causing an increase in the numbers and effectiveness of microbe-killing cells. It also increases production of a chemical, cathelicidin, which kills bacteria. In contrast, active vitamin D damps down the adaptive immune system, particularly any overreactivity to the body's own tissues that could result in damage. Diseases caused by this overactivity, where the immune system attacks its own tissues, are called autoimmune diseases.

What does this mean for infection?

We know from experimental studies in cells or laboratory animals that vitamin D affects the immune system. But what does this mean for infection in people?

Tuberculosis (TB) is one of the most common causes of death from infection worldwide. TB is caused by bacteria that survive within cells of the immune system, relatively hidden from attack by antibodies. In laboratory studies, however, vitamin D-related chemicals (cathelicidin) are produced inside immune cells and these can destroy the TB bacteria. As early as the 1800s people were using cod liver oil or sun exposure to treat TB. Around the middle of the 20th century these natural remedies were replaced by antibiotics, but in the last decade there has been renewed interest in vitamin D, particularly in combination with antibiotics. Unfortunately, while some evidence suggests that vitamin D supplementation might help in the treatment of TB, the results are inconsistent. At this stage there is not enough high-quality evidence to either confirm or deny benefits of vitamin D for TB treatment.

The story is similar for upper respiratory tract infections (URTI), usually caused by either the common cold virus or the influenza virus. We all know that influenza and colds are more common in winter. This is just the time when vitamin D is at its lowest (because of low levels of sun exposure to the skin). But while it is possible that low vitamin D is responsible for the increase in URTI in winter, there are other plausible explanations.

Studies comparing 25D levels in people who do and don't get URTI show that people with lower vitamin D are at higher risk of URTI. However, this could simply be because people with lower vitamin D are more likely to be spending lots of time indoors and exposed to viruses from other people close by. As discussed above, the way to get a clearer idea of whether this is really a vitamin D effect is to randomly assign people to get a vitamin D supplement or placebo then follow them over time to see how many URTI occur in each group.

As with TB, so far these trials have generated inconsistent results, with some trials suggesting that vitamin D might reduce the risk of URTI but others finding no effect. It is difficult to draw any conclusions across all the studies because they have been carried out in different populations (e.g. in old people versus children), using different doses of vitamin D and different ways of measuring whether people have an URTI. To decide whether vitamin D supplementation is really helpful for reducing influenza or the common cold, we need more rigorously conducted randomised trials.

What does this mean for autoimmune diseases?

In autoimmune diseases, the immune system attacks the body's own tissues. In multiple sclerosis (MS), cells of the central nervous system (the brain and spinal cord) are damaged. In type 1 diabetes (T1D), it is the insulin-producing cells in the pancreas that are compromised.

For other autoimmune diseases there is also a specific cell type that is, for some reason, targeted and destroyed by the immune system as though it were a foreign or invading biological threat such as a bacteria or virus. We do not fully understand why this happens. However, active vitamin D specifically acts to suppress or damp down exactly this type of overreactivity, by both depressing the overreactive cells and stimulating regulatory immune cells. These actions provide a believable theory about why vitamin D deficiency may increase the risks of some types of autoimmune diseases, such as MS, T1D, systemic lupus erythematosus and rheumatoid arthritis.

Multiple sclerosis

In the early 1920s it was noticed that MS was more common in people who were born further away from the equator. Later studies showed that people who reported lower levels of past sun exposure also had a higher risk of developing MS. More recent studies have measured 25D levels and shown that lower levels are linked to higher risk of developing MS and of having more severe disease. One challenge with studies in MS is that it is not clear when the disease process actually starts, so that it is not clear at what age the low vitamin D or low sun exposure is most important. However, studies are now underway to test whether vitamin D supplementation (in tablet form), can decrease the risk of developing MS in those who are at high risk.

Type 1 diabetes

Some, but not all, studies have similarly shown that T1D is more common with increasing distance from the equator. T1D is caused by the specific type of immune overreactivity that can be damped down by the active form of vitamin D. This means that there is a plausible pathway from vitamin D deficiency to increased risk of disease. However, studies of vitamin D supplementation in children at higher risk (e.g. those with a family member with T1D) have not been successful in preventing the onset of the disease.

Other autoimmune diseases

For other autoimmune disorders, such as systemic lupus erythematosus and rheumatoid arthritis, there are several studies showing that people with these diseases have lower 25D levels and that the levels are lower in those with more severe disease than in those with less severe disease. However, it is difficult to be clear about whether having severe disease causes people to be outdoors less, thus having lower sun exposure and lower 25D levels, or whether the low 25D levels really are causing the more severe disease. The only way to resolve this uncertainty is through randomised trials to test whether people who are given a vitamin D supplement have lower risk of developing the disease, or have less severe disease, than those given an inactive tablet (placebo). Some such studies are now underway.

What about mental health? Does vitamin D make you feel happier?

Receptors that are activated by vitamin D are present throughout the brain. Studies in animals show that vitamin D deficiency can have negative effects on the brain, including alterations in brain structure and increased anxiety. There is some limited evidence that low 25D levels in pregnancy are linked to an increased risk of autistic tendencies in children and that vitamin D supplementation during pregnancy and infancy is linked to a reduced risk of schizophrenia in adulthood.

Some studies have found that vitamin D deficiency is more common in people with major depression, mood disorders and psychosis, but it is difficult to be sure which came first – the vitamin D deficiency causing the mental health disorder, or the mental health disorder causing lower sun exposure and thus vitamin D deficiency. Again, clinical trials of vitamin D supplementation, testing whether supplementation is better than a placebo, are required to answer this question. Vitamin D supplementation in combination with calcium or an anti-depressant may improve depressive symptoms in groups with major depression, but there is little evidence of an effect of vitamin D alone. Vitamin D supplementation of groups without depression at the start of the study does not seem to be effective in preventing the development of depressive symptoms.

Defying death: do people with higher vitamin D live longer?

Most of us would like to live healthier lives for longer. Can vitamin D help us to do that? The simple answer is that we don't yet know for sure. Several studies show that people with lower 25D levels are at increased risk of dying at a younger age. However, as discussed above, we do not know whether the low vitamin D is the cause of the increased risk or simply a marker of other risk factors for ill health that themselves increase the risk of death.

Again, large randomised trials might be able to give an answer. Several are underway around the world but their results will not be available for some years. Combining the results of many small trials, which were not established specifically to examine death, suggests that there may be a small reduction in the risk of death within a particular timeframe in people who have been supplemented with vitamin D. However, the doses of vitamin D used and the populations studied have been very variable.

At the moment it is not clear whether members of the general population should take a supplement to reduce their risk of earlier death. One interesting study showed that people who had a genetic predisposition to long lives (with relatives who had lived beyond 90 years) actually tended to have lower 25D levels than others of a similar age.

What should my vitamin D level be?

This is a very difficult and highly controversial question. To arrive at an appropriate target 25D level we need to find the level that optimises health. This is made challenging by the measurement issues described earlier, the lack of consensus about which disease conditions are related to vitamin D and the lack of consistency among the many studies. It is also possible that what is 'normal' for one person is not the same as 'normal' in another person.

In 2011, the Institute of Medicine in the USA published a review of the available evidence. The authors concluded that bone health is the only condition for which a causal relation has been established and that a 25D level of 50 nmol/L should be sufficient for the majority of the population. This has been challenged: some scientists and clinicians argue that a level of 75 nmol/L is required but others contend there is not enough evidence for that claim. Currently, Osteoporosis Australia and the Australian and New Zealand Bone and Mineral Society support the IOM conclusion that 50 nmol/L of 25D is required for bone health. They also suggest that aiming for a slightly higher level at the end of summer is necessary to ensure that a level of 50 nmol/L is maintained through most of winter.

What if vitamin D is important for other diseases, and isn't just a marker of lifestyle or health status? Can we work out how much vitamin D we would need in order to make our risk as low as possible? Not really. The challenges of measurement and the highly variable results from different studies make it extraordinarily difficult to decide on a single level that we should have to lower our disease risk (see Table 8.1).

There is, however, general consensus that a level of 30 nmol/L of 25D or lower is clearly deficient and should be treated with vitamin D supplementation. So this is an agreed mark of vitamin D deficiency. Levels between 30 nmol/L and 50 nmol/L may be considered insufficient but there remains debate about whether any specific health problems are likely to be caused by these lower, but probably not dangerously low, levels of 25D.

Table 8.1: Simplified summary of 25D levels and their health implications

25D level	Description	Implications and action
0–30 nmol/L	Deficient	This level is universally accepted as having not enough vitamin D and justifies medical intervention. Discuss treatment with your doctor
31–49 nmol/L	Insufficient	There is debate about what (if any) adverse effects are linked to this level of 25D. It may be normal in mid to late winter. It may be a concern if in late summer
50–100 nmolL	Healthy	This is the range most would agree is healthy. No action is needed
100+ nmol/L	Excessive	Too much vitamin D can be a problem. Discuss this with your doctor. If you are using supplements it may be wise to reduce the dose

Given the uncertainty, what should we do? For the moment, it is probably best to aim for a level of at least 50 nmol/L but lower than 100 nmol/L. There are many scientists working hard to unlock the secrets of vitamin D, and this recommendation may change.

Are there adverse effects from too much vitamin D?

If a little bit is good, isn't more better? In the case of vitamin D, and in fact many other vitamins and minerals, this is not necessarily the case. Studies have suggested that levels of vitamin D that are too high might increase risks of conditions such as prostate cancer, cardiovascular disease, schizophrenia, tuberculosis, babies that are small for their gestational age, and premature death. The problem lies in defining 'too high'. We need more data to work out the optimal range of 25D at both the upper and the lower ends. Until this information is available, it is probably best to err on the side of caution and aim for a moderate level (50–100 nmol/L) of 25D in the bloodstream.

Australia, the sunny country. Surely vitamin D is not a problem for us?

The number of people classified as vitamin D deficient in Australia depends on what level of 25D is used as the cut-off point to define vitamin D deficiency. Obviously the higher the cut-off, the greater the number of people classified as deficient or 'insufficient'. Another difficulty is the problem with vitamin D tests identified above – if the test provides a lower reading than the true value, then more people will be labelled as vitamin D deficient or insufficient. And finally, there are challenges in obtaining blood samples to assess vitamin D status in a group of people that are representative of the population.

While there have been lots of studies in specific subgroups of the population, there are currently only two that give any sort of indication of the level of deficiency in the general population. One, called the AusDiab Study, included ~11 000 people aged 25 and over, who were randomly selected from the population and gave blood samples in 1999–2000. Only 4% of the population had deficient 25D levels (<25 nmol/L) but ~30% of people had a level below 50 nmol/L.

The proportion of the sample who were vitamin D deficient varied by multiple factors including the age and sex of the participants, and the season in which the blood was taken. For example, only 22% of men had a level of <50 nmol/L, compared with 39% of women. In summer 5% of men and 18% of women had a reading below 50 nmol/L compared with 28% of men and 50% of women who were tested in winter. Also, the test used was one that often provides low readings.

In April 2014 the Australian Bureau of Statistics released the 25D results from the Australian Health Survey. This provided a summary of 25D levels in ~10 000 Australians aged 12 years and older who were randomly selected from the Australian population. It is one of the first national surveys in the world that used a vitamin D test that was standardised to the reference measurement protocol developed in the USA, and thus provides definitive results on 25D levels in the Australian population (see Table 8.2).

The results from the National Health Survey showed that, overall, most Australians had sufficient 25D levels; around 7% of Australians had very high or very low levels. As expected

Table 8.2: Vitamin D status of the Australian population*

	Male	Female
Adequate levels: 50 to <100 nmol/L	5637.1 (68.2%)	5872.6 (69.3%)
Mild deficiency: 30–<50 nmol/L	1492.1 (18.1%)	1407.1 (16.6%)
Moderate/severe deficiency: <30 nmol/L	545.2 (6.6%)	556.4 (6.6%)
Excessive levels: >100 nmol/L	592.1 (7.2%)	637.6 (7.5%)

*estimates of persons (thousands), proportions are of the total where results were reported
ABS Survey 2011/12 National Health Survey. % by gender.

vitamin D deficiency was more common in winter and in the southern states, with nearly 50% of people sampled in Victoria and the ACT having levels below 50 nmol/L in winter. Around 60% of Australians who were born overseas in South-East or North-East Asia had inadequate levels; this was nearly 70% for those born in Southern and Central Asia. Although the elderly are generally considered to be an 'at risk' group for vitamin D deficiency, the results of the Australian Health Survey highlight that vitamin D deficiency is most common in the 18–34 years age group (~30% less than 50 nmol/L).

How do I ensure that I get enough vitamin D?

Vitamin D from the sun

Vitamin D is made in the skin following exposure only to the shorter (UVB) wavelengths of solar radiation. As illustrated in Chapter 2, UVB radiation is largely filtered out on its way from the sun to Earth by ozone in our outer atmosphere (the stratosphere). When the sun is low in the sky, UV radiation traverses a longer path through the atmosphere and more UVB is filtered out. When the sun is high in the sky, the path is shorter, and more UVB is present at the Earth's surface. This means that UVB levels are highest in the middle of the day, during summer and at lower latitudes (closer to the equator), and this is when and where vitamin D is made most efficiently.

UVB does not pass through most types of glass. This means that the amount of time we are outdoors is critical to how much vitamin D we make, after taking account of the time of day, time of year and location. Similarly, UVB does not penetrate well through most clothing (see Chapter 4) – vitamin D synthesis increases according to how much skin is directly exposed to the sun.

There is conflicting evidence on how much darker skin pigmentation limits the efficiency of vitamin D synthesis. Darker-skinned people do make vitamin D from sun exposure, but it may take longer to make the same amount as a fairer-skinned person. Although darker-skinned populations often have lower 25D levels than their fairer counterparts, at least some of this is accounted for by cultural differences in sun exposure behaviour and clothing, such as a preference for fairer skin and clothing that covers the arms and legs. Skin pigmentation is a result of the amount of melanin in the outer layer of the skin (the epidermis). Melanin absorbs UVB, so it seems logical that darker skin should require a higher dose of UVB to make vitamin D, but not all the evidence supports this theory. Further, there is some evidence that not everyone requires the same level of 25D. Black Americans have lower 25D levels, on average, than white Americans, but have higher bone density.

How does adhering to 'Slip Slop Slap' influence vitamin D?

Current recommendations are to use sun protection – Slip [on a shirt], Slop [on sunscreen], Slap [on a hat], Seek [shade] and Slide [on some sunglasses] – when the UV Index is 3 or more. Most sunscreens are primarily UVB-blockers, so should block vitamin D synthesis. However, as pointed out in Chapter 5, most of us apply sunscreen at less than half the thickness used by the manufacturer to derive the SPF rating and we often miss bits of our bodies. In these circumstances, sunscreen may decrease the amount of vitamin D that is made for any amount of sun exposure, but it does not stop vitamin D synthesis completely.

We make vitamin D more quickly when the sun is more intense – but our skin is damaged more quickly too. Some recent research shows that our skin still makes vitamin D when the UV Index is less than 3, it just occurs a bit more slowly.

What's the bottom line? How much time should I spend outside to make enough vitamin D? Should I wear sunscreen?

We can take advantage of some of the factors mentioned above to maximise production of vitamin D but minimise the risks of too much sun exposure. Adverse effects of sun exposure mainly affect the head and neck – skin cancers are most common there, and cataracts affect the eyes. Wearing a hat and sunglasses and applying sunscreen helps to protect these areas. Because they are a relatively small skin surface area, they do not contribute very much to vitamin D production. As explained in Chapter 1, skin cancer development is related to DNA damage which is, in turn, related to the dose of UV radiation received by the relevant skin cells. Vitamin D synthesis is summative – i.e. each area of skin that is exposed to the sun contributes to the total vitamin D that is made. So, exposing more skin for a shorter time should maximise vitamin D production but minimise DNA damage in any specific area of skin.

There is some evidence to suggest that prolonged sun exposure results in a plateau of vitamin D production; it doesn't just keep increasing. This is due to a balance being reached between production and destruction of vitamin D. So, shorter but more frequent periods outdoors are preferable to prolonged periods, e.g. sunbaking.

It is difficult to know precisely how much time we need to spend in the sun. It would vary with the amount of skin exposed, the time of year (less in summer than winter), location (less in the north of Australia than the south) and skin colour (less for fairer- than for darker-skinned people). There are some guidelines, e.g. http://www.cancer.org.au/preventing-cancer/sun-protection/vitamin-d/how-much-sun-is-enough.html.

These are based on calculations that combine information on the usual levels of UV radiation that reach Earth's surface with information from experiments that used sunbeds to deliver UV radiation. We don't really know how well these experiments relate to our everyday lives, so the guidelines may change as more information becomes available. It is important to clarify that we are not recommending the use of sunbeds to boost vitamin D! Chapter 3 covers the issue of sunbeds and the dangers they pose.

Vitamin D from food and supplements

The alternative to getting vitamin D from exposure to the sun is to ingest it in food or supplements. The current Australian recommendations for people who have minimal sun exposure vary according to age. People under 50 years old should consume 200 IU/day; people aged 51–70 and those who are over 70 should consume 400 IU/day and 600 IU/day respectively. However, these amounts may be insufficient to ensure that people have a 25D level of 50 nmol/L if they have no sun exposure. The US Institute of Medicine has estimated that, to achieve this level in the complete absence of sun exposure, people under 70 should ingest 600 IU/day and those over 70 should consume 800 IU/day.

The best food sources of vitamin D are oily fish such as salmon. One small piece of salmon (100 g) contains ~360 IU but most people don't eat salmon very often. Some milk in Australia is fortified with vitamin D but most fortified milks contain only ~50 IU in a 250 mL glass. All margarine and dairy blend spreads in Australia are fortified but one tablespoon of margarine contains only ~60 IU of vitamin D, so you would need to eat a lot to reach the recommended daily intake!

There are many supplements available without prescription in Australia. Some multivitamins contain vitamin D. Alternatively, there are tablets that contain only vitamin D or that contain vitamin D and calcium.

The sun causes skin cancer – why don't I just take a supplement?

Exposing our skin to the sun increases the risk of skin cancer, and Australia is the skin cancer capital of the world. So maybe we should all avoid the sun as much as possible and just take a vitamin D supplement to ensure sufficient vitamin D status. Unfortunately, it may not be that simple. There is some evidence that not all the beneficial effects of sun exposure come through vitamin D. There may be other pathways whereby sun exposure makes us feel better and improves our health. For the moment, then, the recommendation is for careful sun exposure, rather than sun avoidance with vitamin D supplementation.

Conclusion

Severe vitamin D deficiency causes rickets in children and osteomalacia in adults. It can cause muscle pain and weakness, and may contribute to osteoporosis. In conjunction with calcium, vitamin D supplementation can decrease the risk of falls and fractures in the elderly. Despite considerable research linking vitamin D deficiency to increased risk of a range of diseases, clinical trials of vitamin D supplementation have not provided convincing evidence of beneficial effects.

It has been difficult to define target optimal 25D levels, due to the challenges of wide variation in the accuracy of vitamin D tests and the lack of a suitable outcome against which to calibrate 'optimal'. Widespread vitamin D deficiency is reported, but without confidence in the accurate measurement of 25D or clear evidence of what level to aim for, we can't be confident that this is a real problem in Australia. International efforts are improving vitamin D tests, but this solves only part of the problem. We still need to define what 'vitamin D deficiency' is, in terms of 25D concentration.

Concerns about vitamin D deficiency have led to confusion about the correct sun protection/sun exposure advice. Australia has the highest skin cancer incidence in the world. To our best knowledge, short (three- to five-minute) exposures to our intense summer sunlight should be sufficient to maintain good vitamin D status. In winter, advice will vary according to location, with longer and more frequent exposure to greater body surface area required in high-latitude regions such as Tasmania. Where this is not feasible (e.g. because the exposure times are too long or it is too cold to expose much skin), vitamin D supplementation may be required. Achieving higher 25D levels by the end of summer will help to maintain adequate vitamin D status during winter.

Further reading

Hewer S, Lucas R, van der Mei I, Taylor BV (2013) Vitamin D and multiple sclerosis. *Journal of Clinical Neuroscience* **20**, 634–641. doi:10.1016/j.jocn.2012.10.005.

Lai JK, Lucas RM, Clements MS, Harrison SL, Banks E (2010) Assessing vitamin D status: pitfalls for the unwary. *Molecular Nutrition and Food Research* **54**, 1062–1071.

Peterlik M (2012) Vitamin D insufficiency and chronic diseases: hype and reality. *Food and Function* **3**, 784–794. doi:10.1039/c2fo10262e.

Ralph AP, Lucas RM, Norval M (2013) Vitamin D and solar ultraviolet radiation in the risk and treatment of tuberculosis. *Lancet Infectious Diseases* **13**, 77–88. doi:10.1016/S1473-3099(12)70275-X.

Rosen CJ, Taylor CL (2013) Common misconceptions about vitamin D: implications for clinicians. *Nature Reviews. Endocrinology* **9**, 434–438. doi:10.1038/nrendo.2013.75.

Chapter 9

Early detection saves lives: what should we look for?

Jon Emery

Key messages

- A skin cancer that is identified and treated in the early stages of development is more likely to be treated successfully and leave less scarring and long-term damage.
- A checklist that is commonly used to help people identify a 'suspicious' lesion or skin problem that may be melanoma is the ABCDE system.
- People should look for a skin spot that is **A**symmetrical, has an irregular **B**order, has different **C**olours, has an enlarging **D**iameter or is **E**volving or changing in some way.
- General medical practitioners (GPs) are the best source of advice in first identifying and often managing any possible skin cancers. Those who have trained or carried out most of their practice in Australia are likely to be experienced in skin cancer, because it is so common.
- Where appropriate, GPs will refer people with skin cancer problems to specialist doctors.

Like most cancers, the earlier skin cancer is found and treated, the better the chance of preventing the cancer spreading and causing serious illness or death. This is very much the case for melanoma but it also applies to non-melanoma skin cancer and specifically squamous cell carcinoma (SCC), which currently causes more than 400 deaths in Australia each year.

Table 9.1: Proportion of people who survive at least five years after diagnosis, by stage of melanoma

Stage at diagnosis	5-year survival (%)
IA	97
IB	92
IIA	81
IIB	70
IIC	53
IIIA	78
IIIB	59
IIIC	40
IV	15–20

Early detection of skin cancer is important; for non-melanoma skin cancers this may mean simpler, less disfiguring treatments. For melanoma, the earlier it is diagnosed, the more likely that it can be cured. Table 9.1 shows how the chances of surviving at least five years after diagnosis vary by 'stage', based on an assessment of the melanoma's thickness, whether it is ulcerated and how much it had spread by the time of diagnosis.

How do we identify 'suspicious' lesions?

Diagnosing skin cancer is not simple, so doctors look for features that make them more suspicious that a lesion may be cancerous.

The following are features to look out for with basal cell carcinomas (BCCs), the commonest and least serious skin cancer (see Figs 9.1, 9.2, 9.3):

- a red, pale or pearly patch of skin;
- a lump or scaly area which fails to heal;
- slow-growing over months to years;
- usually on areas of sun exposure such as the face, ears and forearms.

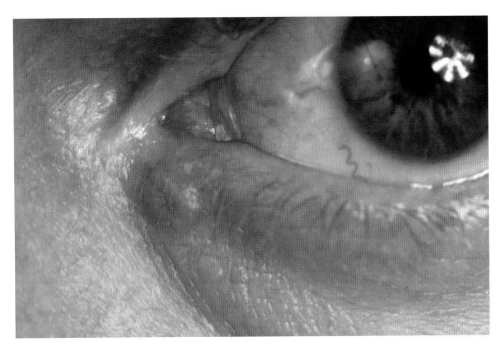

Fig. 9.1: Basal cell carcinoma.

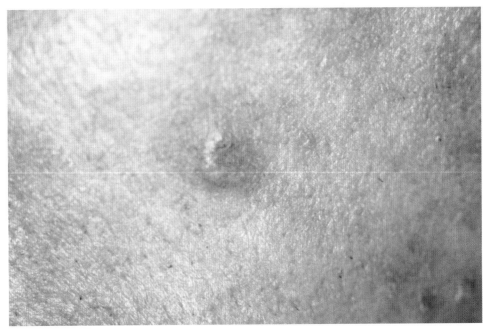

Fig. 9.2: Basal cell carcinoma on the face. Note the slightly pearl-like surface. Image supplied by Dr Carl Vinciullo.

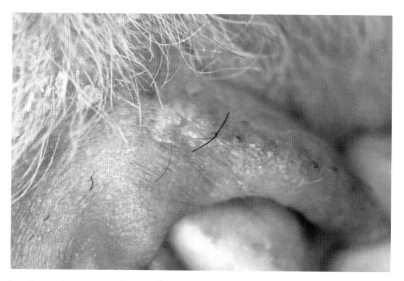

Fig. 9.3: Basal cell carcinoma on the ear lobe. Image supplied by Dr Carl Vinciullo.

SCCs have the following features, some of which overlap with BCCs (see Figs 9.4, 9.5):

- a thickened red area of skin, sometimes with a central depressed area;
- have a crust and bleed easily;
- slow-growing over months;
- usually on areas of sun exposure such as lips, ears, bald scalp and forearms.

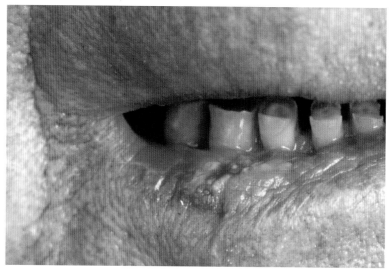

Fig. 9.4: Squamous cell carcinoma on the lip. Note the ulceration.

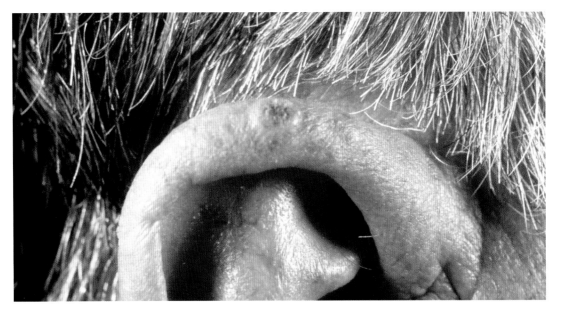

Fig. 9.5: Squamous cell carcinoma on the ear. Image supplied by Dr Carl Vinciullo.

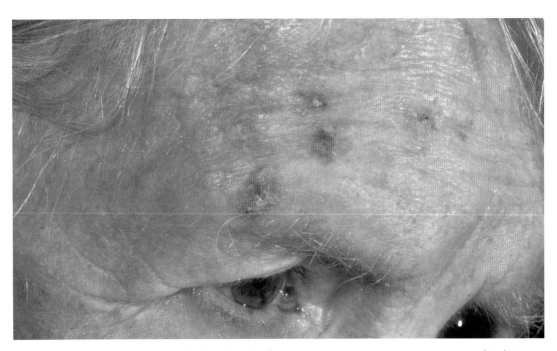

Fig. 9.6: Solar keratosis on the forehead. Solar keratosis is a common non-cancerous skin lesion due to long-term sun damage. It is common on the face, scalp and arms and may have features suggestive of basal cell or squamous cell carcinomas.

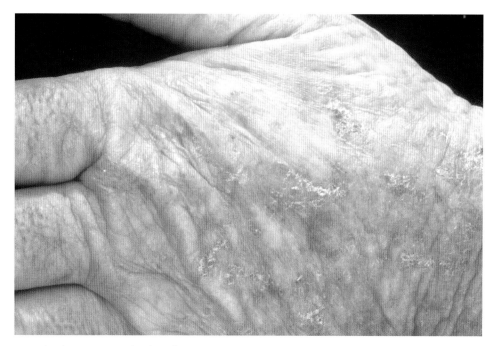

Fig. 9.7: Solar keratosis on the hand.

Melanomas can arise from existing moles or as new lesions. Curiously, they can appear anywhere on your skin, not just on sun-exposed areas, so it is important to look for changes to moles over your whole body, even the soles of your feet. Two checklists have been developed to help identify lesions which are suspicious of melanoma. The first is the ABCDE checklist, developed by the American Cancer Society and American Academy of Dermatology in 1985 to help people review any moles about which they were concerned. For each mole you should run through the following criteria.

A for Asymmetry. If you drew a line through the middle of the mole, would the two halves look the same?

B for Border. Does the mole have an irregular edge?

C for Colour. Does the mole have areas of different colours such as black, blue or red, white or grey?

D for Diameter. Is the mole more than 6 mm in diameter?

E for Evolving. Is the mole changing in size, shape or colour?

The second checklist to help assess moles is the seven-point checklist (7-PC) devised by a group of dermatologists in Glasgow for use both by ordinary people and GPs. The features in the 7-PC are:

- change in size of lesion;
- irregular pigmentation or colour;
- irregular border;
- inflammation;
- itch or altered sensation;
- larger than other lesions (diameter >7 mm);
- oozing or crusting of lesion.

A later version developed a scoring system so that change in size, irregular colour and irregular border each scored two points, and the other features scored one point each. A combined score of three or more was said to identify suspicious lesions, although research we have recently published suggests a cut-off score of four may be more accurate in general practice. An Australian study comparing use of the ABCDE and 7-PC checklists by consumers found that changes in size and colour were the most important features in helping distinguish melanoma from benign lesions.

It is important to realise that many benign lesions will show some features of the ABCDE and 7-PC checklists (see Figs 9.8–9.15). They are not always a sign of skin cancer. Your doctor will assess any changes you may notice and advise what needs to be done. In some cases the lesions may be safe to leave untreated, in other cases they may need to be treated or removed.

There is one other rule which can be applied to help identify moles suspicious of melanoma – the delightfully named 'ugly duckling' sign. The idea is to compare all your moles. If one or more looks very different from all the others, i.e. is an 'ugly duckling', this is suspicious and should be reviewed by a doctor.

It is therefore important to be aware of these various features of skin cancer and keep an eye out when you are showering, for any changes to your skin. Obviously, checking certain areas of your body such as your back can be difficult. You may want to use a hand mirror to help or ask your partner to have a look. Quite often, concerns about a mole identified by a partner, relative or friend prompt patients to actually get it checked by a doctor.

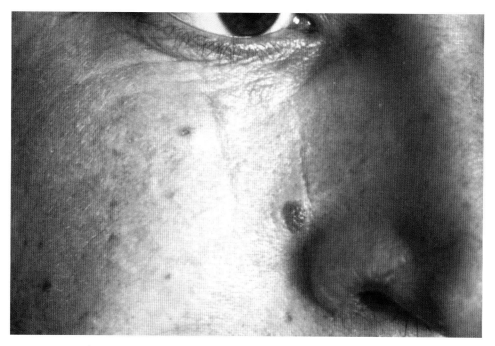

Fig. 9.8: Compound naevus. This is a benign mole. Note its regular shape, border and colour.

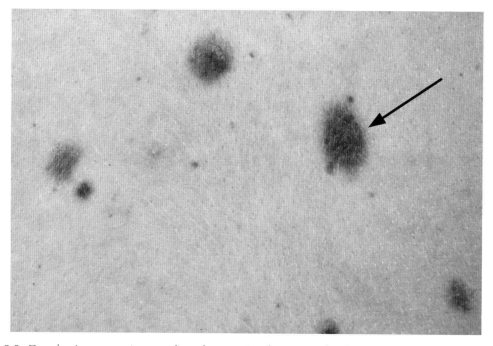

Fig. 9.9: Dysplastic naevus (arrowed) and some simple naevi. The dysplastic naevus is larger with an irregular border.

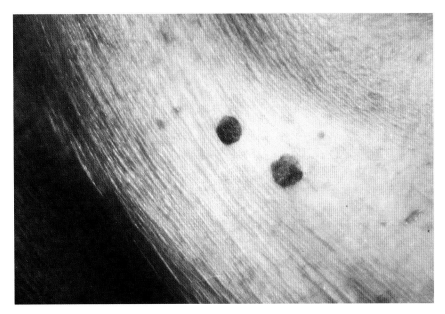

Fig. 9.10: Seborrhoeic keratosis. Note the slightly raised warty appearance. These are often mistaken for melanomas because of their irregular colour and large size.

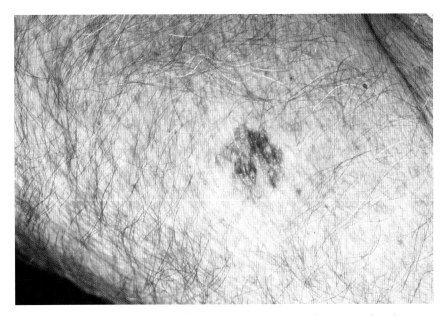

Fig. 9.11: Lentigo maligna. This is a type of precursor to the development of melanoma or very early melanoma which has not started to invade the skin. It is usually seen on badly sun-damaged skin such as the face in elderly people. Note it has several features suggestive of melanoma, such as irregular shape, border and colour.

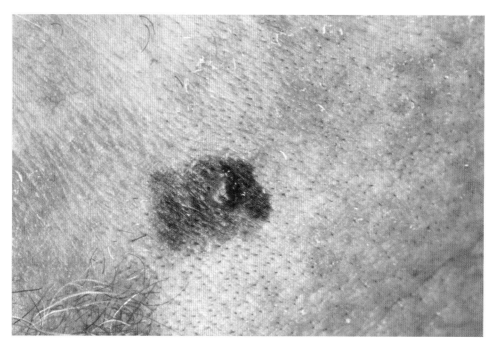

Fig. 9.12: Melanoma on the face. Note the asymmetry (A), irregular border (B) and colour (C) with a central raised area. Image supplied by Dr Carl Vinciullo.

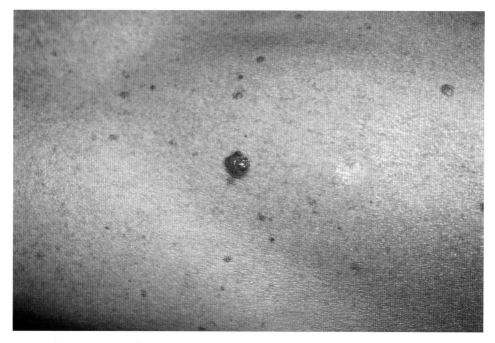

Fig. 9.13: Melanoma. Note the irregular border (B) and colour (C). Image supplied by Dr Carl Vinciullo.

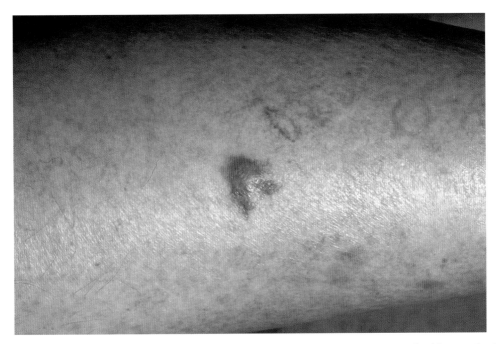

Fig. 9.14: Melanoma. Note the irregular border (B) and colour (C). Image supplied by Dr Carl Vinciullo.

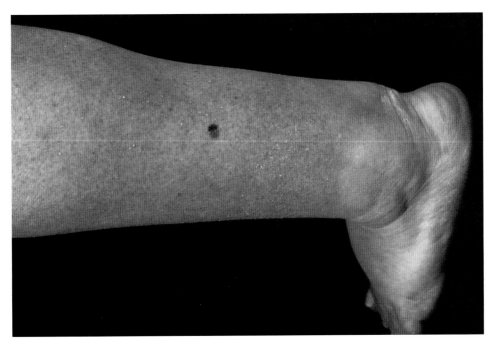

Fig. 9.15: Melanoma. Note the asymmetry (A) and irregular colour (C).

Seeing a doctor about suspicious lesions

When you go to a doctor with concerns about a skin lesion, they will probably ask questions in the following areas:

- changes you have noticed in specific skin lesions;
- any previous skin cancers in you or your close relatives;
- your history of sun exposure and use of preventive measures;
- other medical conditions which may increase your risk of skin cancer, such as immunosuppressant drugs.

The doctor will then examine your skin, starting with the lesion you are concerned about, and then possibly the rest of your body. Some doctors will use additional tools to help assess your moles. For example, they may use a dermatoscope (see Fig. 9.16), a hand-held tool which looks similar to the device they use to examine your ears. It is a magnifying lens which, when used with a small amount of oil on the surface of the skin lesion, allows specific features to be seen which are not visible by the naked eye. The doctor must be trained in interpreting these features but it can be a useful additional tool in identifying suspicious lesions. Some clinics will use a computerised dermatoscope

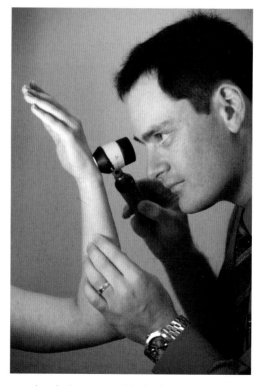

Fig. 9.16: A dermatoscope used to help assess skin lesions.

which allows higher-level magnification and, more importantly, the digital storage of images. This allows lesions to be monitored over time. If a lesion has not changed over a three- to six-month period, it is very unlikely to be skin cancer and can therefore be safely left alone.

'If in doubt, cut it out'?

When the doctor examines the skin lesion, they will be applying similar rules to those in the checklists described above to determine the likelihood that it is skin cancer and which type it might be. This will help determine one of three options:

- no suspicion of skin cancer, so leave alone and ask the patient to return if any further changes are noticed;
- intermediate level of suspicion, so ask the patient to monitor and return in three months for review. This might involve trying to obtain a photo of the lesion, or storing a dermoscopy image on the computer for subsequent comparison;
- high level of suspicion, so cut the lesion out or refer the patient to a specialist.

Some people may wonder why doctors do not simply remove everything, even if it is very unlikely to be skin cancer. There are several reasons: even apparently simple surgery involves small risks such as infection and pain, and surgery inevitably leaves a scar, however skilled the surgeon.

There are financial considerations too: you may have out-of-pocket expenses for the procedure itself and, perhaps more significantly from the taxpayer perspective, excisions of benign or harmless skin lesions are a major cost to Medicare. In 2010 $93.5 million was spent by Medicare on the treatment of non-melanoma skin cancer and this figure is rising year by year. This amount does not account for the large number of excisions performed on harmless skin lesions. Your Medicare dollar may be better spent elsewhere than on removing lesions which are very clearly benign or which can be safely monitored for change. And avoiding unnecessary surgery lessens the out-of-pocket costs.

How good are GPs at diagnosing skin cancer and would I do better to go to a skin cancer clinic?

GPs in Australia are trained to manage a very wide range of conditions including the assessment of possible skin cancers. It is very reasonable to see your regular GP if you have concerns about a skin lesion. There is an alternative option, to attend a primary-care skin cancer clinic. The doctors in these clinics are usually GPs who have decided to focus on skin cancer and who can be seen without requiring a referral to a specialist skin doctor such as a dermatologist or plastic surgeon. Skin cancer clinics are more likely to use dermoscopy and computer storage of images, allowing computerised monitoring of lesions. The question is, are they more accurate at diagnosing skin cancer than regular GPs?

There have been several studies, mainly conducted in Queensland, which have examined the accuracy of doctors at diagnosing skin cancer in regular general practice and in primary-care skin cancer clinics. There are various measures used to assess this. One such measure is the 'number needed to excise' (NNE) – the number of skin lesions removed per one diagnosis of skin cancer. It is therefore a reflection of how accurate the doctor is at picking skin cancers from benign lesions. In the largest study in Queensland, it was shown that the NNE to diagnose any type of skin cancer was two for both GPs and skin cancer clinics. In other words, they get it right ~50% of the time. However, the figures are quite different for melanoma. The NNE for melanoma is 20 and is the same for GPs and skin cancer clinic doctors. This means they get it right ~5% of the time. This may sound pretty terrible but it is a reflection of how difficult diagnosing melanoma can be. It also suggests a relatively low threshold to cutting out a lesion when there is some degree of suspicion. Given the potential seriousness of melanoma, this is very reasonable.

Do I need regular skin checks?

Skin cancer clinics and some GPs may promote regular full-body examinations of your skin even if you have not noticed any particular changes. This type of skin cancer screening remains controversial, just like other types of cancer screening such as for prostate cancer. One of the reasons for this controversy is that there have been no trials which show that screening people who are at average risk of developing melanoma actually makes any difference to their chances of dying from melanoma. It may be that all we are doing is removing lots of skin lesions, including some very early melanomas, which would not have caused any harm or would have been detected anyway when symptoms developed. Also, you will incur more costs to yourself and Medicare for a potentially unnecessary examination and/or skin excision.

Current national guidance by expert groups, such as the National Health and Medical Research Council, does not recommend regular full-body skin examinations unless you are at very high risk of melanoma, e.g. because of a previous diagnosis of melanoma or a very strong family history of melanoma. Because of these controversies, the most important thing to do is to become familiar with your skin and be aware of any changes.

When do I need a referral to a specialist?

GPs vary in what they feel competent at managing themselves, and what they choose to refer. Some GPs have had additional specific training in dermatology or minor surgery and may therefore manage more complex skin lesions. Other GPs may choose to refer for a specialist opinion. Dermatologists are highly specialised experts in all skin conditions and are very skilled at assessing lesions which may be cancerous. Thus, you may be referred to a dermatologist if there is greater uncertainty about a diagnosis. People who are at increased risk of melanoma due to a strong family history of the condition may require regular examination of their skin and monitoring of skin lesions. Again, this is something that may be better offered by a dermatologist.

As well as a GP's level of expertise, there are other factors that determine decisions about referral. The size and location of the lesion is important, particularly if it is on the face. A referral to a plastic surgeon may well be warranted in these circumstances. They are experts at performing dermatological surgery; if the lesion is in a location or of a size which requires more complex surgery, a plastic surgeon may be best suited.

GPs often perform the initial excision of a mole suspected to be a melanoma. Such an excision would usually take a very small amount of surrounding normal skin. If a melanoma is diagnosed, this requires a wider excision of skin surrounding the melanoma. Because skin cancer cells grow and spread, removal of skin around the lesion is necessary to take away possible cancer cells that might have started to spread but that are not yet visible to the naked eye. If successful, this reduces the chance of the cancer continuing to grow and spread to other parts of the skin or body. Requiring a wider skin excision after the initial diagnosis of melanoma is another reason for referral to a specialist. It also allows discussion with a specialist about the detailed pathological findings of the melanoma and requirements for further treatment and follow-up.

New technologies in melanoma diagnosis

Given the evidence about the challenges of accurately diagnosing this type of skin cancer, one of the 'holy grails' of research in melanoma is developing new technologies to improve diagnosis.

The strongest evidence is still for dermoscopy as a diagnostic aid but, as mentioned already, this technique requires significant training and practice for proficiency. Various other imaging techniques are at different stages of development. Their role in supporting better diagnosis, particularly in general practice, remains uncertain. For example, a trial of a device called Molemate using a method called siascopy found that it was no better than getting GPs to systematically use the 7-PC.

Perhaps the biggest growth area at present is the use of smartphone technology to help consumers assess their own moles. A review of melanoma apps published in 2012 found 26 different applications available for use on a smartphone; no doubt there will be more than this by the time you read this book. Some apps allow a dermatoscope to be attached to a smartphone, although these are intended primarily for doctors because of the difficulty of interpreting the images.

Several apps allow a consumer to take a photo of a skin lesion; in some cases the image can be sent to a dermatologist to review (for a fee). Alternatively, the app will conduct an automatic analysis of the lesion, usually evaluating it using the ABCDE criteria. There is limited evidence about the accuracy of these types of app.

Another type of app allows consumers to monitor their own skin lesions. The smartphone takes a photo of the lesion and the app stores the image, sending reminders at specified periods to take another photo. This may be useful in identifying change in key features such as colour, size and shape. Evidence for the usefulness of this approach remains to be shown and so it is probably too early to recommend them.

In the meantime, GPs in Australia remain the most effective 'front line' in the diagnosis and management of skin cancer. Because skin cancer is so common in this country, most GPs have considerable experience and success in diagnosing skin cancer early.

Further reading

American Academy of Dermatology. www.aad.org/spot-skin-cancer/understanding-skin-cancer/ how-do-i-check-my-skin/what-to-look-for.

Cancer Council Victoria. www.cancervic.org.au/about-cancer/cancer_types/skin_cancers_non_ melanoma&utm_source=google&utm_medium=cpc&utm_content=Skin-cancer&utm_ campaign=Cancer-types.

Chapter 10

Melanoma treatment

Judy Cole

Key messages

- The primary treatment for melanoma is surgery.
- A melanoma that is found and treated at the earliest stages of development is more likely to be successfully treated.
- Stages 1 and 2 are early stage melanoma; stages 3 and 4 are more advanced melanoma.
- In all cases doctors aim to ensure they remove all cancer cells at and near the melanoma, and that means they will cut away what might look like healthy skin near the lesion. In addition to surgery, other treatment may be required in some cases and may include chemotherapy and radiotherapy. In other cases, biological or targeted therapies may be needed.
- A person diagnosed with melanoma might consider that other family members may be more susceptible to skin cancer in the future. A conversation with doctors will help guide that discussion.

Early surgery

The treatment for a suspected melanoma is surgical excision. Usually this involves a procedure done under local anaesthetic (an injection to numb the skin) in a day surgery or doctor's office surgery. Wherever possible, suspicious lesions should be completely excised with a small amount of normal-looking skin (~2 mm) from around the margin, often in the shape of an ellipse. The wound is then sutured together. Partial biopsies including shave and punch biopsies may miss some of the abnormal cells and lead to errors in diagnosis, and are therefore not recommended.

The skin specimen (biopsy) that your doctor removes is placed in a small jar containing a preservative (formalin) and sent to a pathology laboratory for analysis by a specialist doctor called a histopathologist. The results are usually available within seven days.

When the histopathologist confirms that you have a melanoma, your doctor will receive a written report (histopathology report). This details the type of melanoma, how many millimetres the melanoma has spread into the skin (Breslow thickness), how deeply the melanoma has gone through the layers of the skin (Clark level, Fig. 10.1) and confirms whether the margins of excision are adequate.

You will generally be asked to return to your doctor for a re-excision, sometimes referred to as 'wide local excision'. This involves removal of more tissue (5–10 mm) from around the scar to ensure that there is an adequate amount of normal skin (a safety margin) around the melanoma site. This second specimen is also sent to the pathology laboratory for analysis to ensure that there are no remaining abnormal cells in the area. The aim is to avoid leaving any abnormal cells that might continue to grow and which could then spread.

After the extra tissue is cut out the wound is sutured together. Sometimes the wound is too large to be sutured together; if so, the doctor may need to use either a skin flap or a skin graft to cover the wound. A skin flap involves pulling over skin nearby and stitching it over the wound. With a

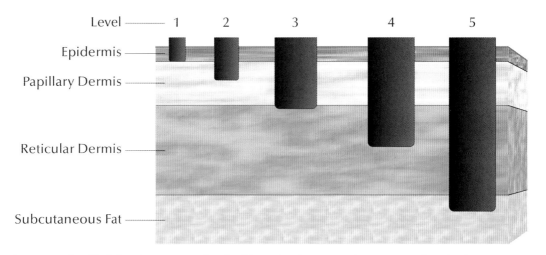

Fig. 10.1: The Clark level measures depth of invasion by anatomic structure. Level 1 is synonymous with an in situ melanoma.

skin graft, skin is taken from another part of the body and placed over the area where the melanoma was removed.

Whatever sort of surgery you have for your melanoma, the wound will be covered with a dressing and checked after a few days to ensure that it is healing well. The wound may be sore for a few days but most of the time simple painkillers like paracetamol will ease the discomfort. The wound will look red immediately after surgery but with time the redness will fade to leave a pale scar.

If your melanoma is detected early this may be all the treatment you need. In Australia, more than 85% of people with melanoma are cured by this early surgery. However, your doctor will still advise that your skin be checked regularly as you may develop a new melanoma somewhere else on the body. People who have had one melanoma have more than five times the risk of developing another melanoma than an average person of their age. At these visits your scar will be checked and the doctor will see if any lymph nodes are enlarged. Lymph nodes form part of the body's lymphatic system (see Fig. 10.2) and act as filters, trapping cancer cells including melanoma.

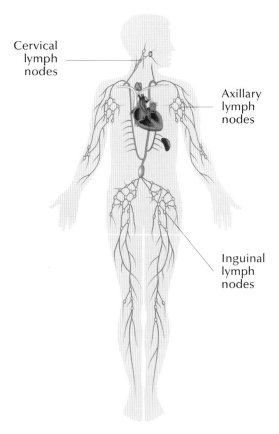

Fig. 10.2: Lymph nodes. Image courtesy WA Department of Health.

Tests to determine if the melanoma has spread

When it is confirmed that you have a melanoma the doctor will need to determine if your melanoma has spread. Melanoma can spread in three ways. It can invade local tissue, spread through the lymphatic system and spread through the blood to other places in the body. Your doctor will examine (feel) the nearby lymph nodes to see if the melanoma has spread. If the lymph nodes feel enlarged, the doctor may recommend a fine needle aspiration (FNA) biopsy. This is where a sample of cells is taken from the enlarged node by inserting a needle and drawing tissue into a syringe. This tissue sample is examined by a histopathologist to see if it contains any melanoma cells.

If the melanoma is very thin, which means the melanoma cells have not spread more than 1 mm into the skin (thin melanoma), you will probably not need any special tests. However, if it is thicker than 1 mm the doctor may talk to you about a sentinel lymph node biopsy (Fig. 10.3). This test has not been shown to improve your outcome but it can give valuable information to your doctor about the likelihood of your melanoma having spread.

The sentinel lymph node is the lymph node that drains the area where the melanoma developed. It can be located and tested to see if the melanoma has spread to the lymphatic system. This technique is called sentinel lymph node biopsy. Melanomas that have spread into the lymphatic system may also be more likely to spread into the blood.

To have a sentinel lymph node biopsy, the doctor will arrange for you to attend a nuclear medicine department where a small amount of radioactive fluid is injected into the skin where the melanoma was removed. This is called lymphoscintigraphy.

The surgery is then performed under a general anaesthetic within a few hours. The surgeon injects a blue dye into the skin around the same site where the melanoma was removed. The blue dye travels to the sentinel node, turning it blue. The surgeon passes a machine called a gamma probe over the area to guide the surgery to the blue radioactive sentinel node. The surgeon then removes this lymph node, stitches up the wound and sends the node to the pathology laboratory for examination. Occasionally there is more than one sentinel node, in which case you may have two or more small wounds.

If melanoma cells are found in the sentinel node, the surgeon will recommend removal of all the other lymph nodes in that area (lymph node dissection). This is a larger operation performed in hospital under a general anaesthetic. It is done to try to stop melanoma coming back in the same area.

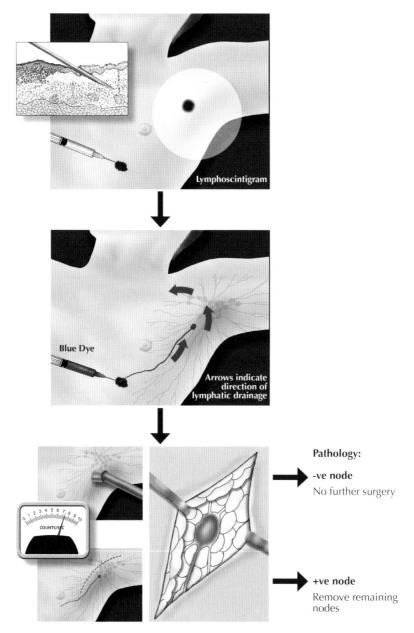

Fig. 10.3: The sentinel node biopsy procedure.

Other tests

Other tests that may be recommended to see if a melanoma has spread include blood tests, CT scans, a PET scan (see Fig. 10.4) and molecular testing of the melanoma.

A CT scan is a Computed Tomography scan, also known as a CAT (Computer Axial Tomography) scan. It is a machine that can form a full three-dimensional computer model of the inside of the body and detect whether a melanoma has spread inside the body to areas like the lungs, liver or brain.

A PET scan (Positron Emission Tomography) is an imaging test that uses a radioactive substance called a tracer to see how far a melanoma has spread. The tracer is given through a vein (intravenous, IV), most often on the inside of your elbow. The tracer travels through the blood and collects in deposits of melanoma in the organs and tissues. This helps the radiologist see certain areas of concern more clearly.

Combined PET/CT machines are used in most centres since combining the scans can create a more complete picture of the body than either test can offer alone.

Molecular testing has recently begun to be performed on melanoma specimens. Genes, which are made up of DNA, act as instructions to make molecules called proteins. Some melanoma cells have a change (mutation) in a gene called BRAF. This gene makes a protein called B-Raf which is involved in sending signals inside cells causing cell growth. This gene signals melanoma cells to multiply. About half the people with melanoma have this gene change in the melanoma. It can be detected by testing melanoma tissue that is removed during surgery. BRAF gene mutation testing has become an important tool for diagnosis, prognosis, treatment and predicting patient outcome in response to targeted therapy.

Other patients with melanoma have a mutation in a gene called KIT. This gene is also involved in cell signalling and multiplication; abnormalities in this gene can lead to growth of melanoma.

Stages of disease

Based on examination of your body and diagnostic tests including biopsy and imaging, the doctor will be able to tell how far your melanoma has grown into the skin and whether it has spread from the skin to the lymph nodes or other parts of the body. This is called staging. The system most often used to stage melanoma is the American Joint Commission on Cancer (AJCC) TNM system – Tumour, Node and Metastases. This staging system describes the size of a primary tumour (T), whether any lymph nodes contain cancer cells (N) and whether the cancer has spread to another part of the body (M). Staging is important because it determines the kind of treatment you need, the likely risk of the melanoma coming back after treatment and whether you need tests to see whether the melanoma has spread.

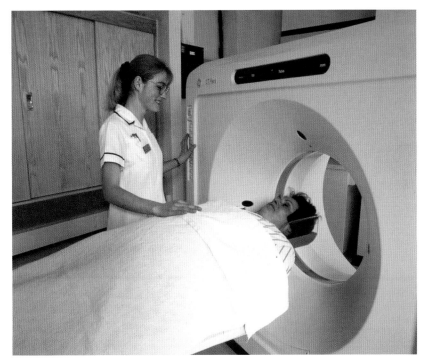

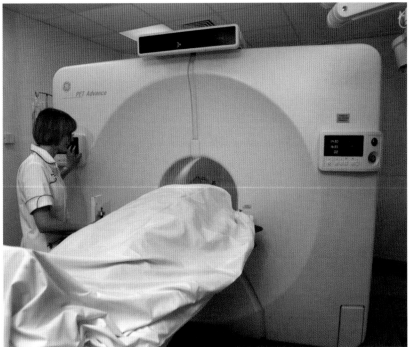

Fig. 10.4: A CT scanning unit and a PET scanning unit, with patient and technician operator. Wellcome Photo Library.

If a melanoma is only in the skin it is called stage 1 or stage 2, depending on how thick it is. These melanomas can very often be cured by surgery without any additional treatment.

If melanoma is found in the lymph system it is called stage 3. Often (but not always) the first place a melanoma heads for is the lymph nodes.

If melanoma is found in other parts of the body away from where the melanoma started it is called stage 4. The most common places are the lungs, liver and brain.

Stages 3 and 4 where melanoma has spread beyond the skin are called advanced melanoma or metastatic melanoma. This type of melanoma is really hard to cure.

The stage of melanoma determines the chances of survival (prognosis) – the expected outcome of your melanoma. The outcome is best if you have stage 1 melanoma and worst if you have stage 4.

Treatment of advanced melanoma

People with advanced melanoma need to be cared for by a range of health professionals who specialise in different aspects of melanoma treatment. This multidisciplinary team may include a medical oncologist who prescribes and coordinates drug treatment, a radiation oncologist who prescribes and coordinates a course of radiation treatment and a specialist nurse who can support you throughout your treatment. Other helpful people include social workers, psychologists, counsellors and dieticians as well as a palliative care team.

In major cities in Australia, patients are sometimes treated by a multidisciplinary team in specialist melanoma centres where the specialists work together, discuss your diagnosis and decide the best plan for your treatment. The specialist doctors will discuss the options with you and your family and decide on the treatment depending on where the melanoma has spread to, the symptoms it is causing and the treatments you have already had.

This may involve several steps.

1   Surgery. Some melanomas that have spread to other parts of the body can be removed by surgery. This is usually possible if the melanoma has spread to other areas on the skin or to the lymph nodes, and sometimes when it has spread to internal organs.

2   Radiation therapy. This uses very powerful energy beams to kill melanoma cells. During treatment you lie on a table under a machine that aims radiation at the affected part of your body. The treatment takes only a few minutes and you don't feel any pain but it needs to be

repeated each day for several weeks. It can be used to control melanoma growth or relieve symptoms when melanoma has spread to other parts of the body.

Radiation therapy can cause side effects, depending on the part of the body that is being treated. The skin in the treatment area may become red and sore and you may feel quite tired during your treatment.

3   Chemotherapy. This involves medicines that kill cancer cells. Unfortunately, chemotherapy can also kill normal cells and this can lead to side effects. There are many different types of chemotherapy, including pills and medicines that are injected straight into the bloodstream. The chemotherapy drugs most commonly used to treat metastatic melanoma are called dacarbazine and fotemustine. Some chemotherapy for melanoma has only mild side effects; more aggressive chemotherapy is often associated with tiredness, poor appetite and low blood counts. Unfortunately chemotherapy is not very effective for most melanoma patients.

If you have melanoma that has returned after initial treatment but is confined to an arm or leg, you may receive chemotherapy just to that area. This is called regional infusion therapy. In this procedure, doctors isolate the affected limb from the rest of the body by stopping blood flow with a tourniquet then expose the limb to high levels of chemotherapy. This maximises the effect of chemotherapy on the tumour, while limiting the side effects on the rest of your body.

4   Biological therapy. This form of treatment helps your immune system fight the melanoma cells. Interferon is a drug that has been used for many years; it can be given into a vein or injected under the skin. It can cause side effects similar to flu symptoms. Interleukin 2 is another drug used in immunotherapy. There have been a lot of developments in this area recently and several new drugs are being used including ipilimumab (marketed as Yervoy®). This drug works by activating the immune system to attack melanoma cells. Ipilimumab is given as a liquid injected into a vein (or infusion) once every three weeks for up to four infusions. Ipilimumab can help some patients with advanced melanoma by shrinking tumours and improving their life expectancy. The most common side effects of ipilimumab include skin rashes, itching and diarrhoea.

5   Targeted therapy. This is a form of treatment in which drugs destroy the melanoma cells while leaving the normal cells in the body intact. The drugs are targeted to the melanoma – they may be more effective and have fewer side effects than chemotherapy and radiation therapy. They are designed to be used by people whose disease has certain molecular characteristics. These drugs include vemurafenib (marketed as Zelboraf®) and dabrafenib (marketed as Tafinlar) and are designed to help patients who have a mutation in a gene called BRAF. The BRAF inhibitor drugs can help to slow or stop melanoma cells from growing. The most

common side effects include joint pain, skin rash and sensitivity to sunlight (vemurafenib) and fever (dabrafenib). A major drawback is that the drugs seem to work for only a limited time before the melanoma starts growing again.

Taking part in a clinical trial

Doctors and researchers continue to look for new ways to improve the treatment for advanced melanoma. New and better treatment options are being sought and, when a promising option is found through laboratory research, it is tested in clinical trials on sufferers. Clinical trials are the only way to establish if a new treatment will work safely and effectively in people.

The doctor may suggest you consider being enrolled in a clinical trial. These are important in developing new treatments for melanoma, in particular to determine whether new treatments are safe and effective and work better than current treatments. Over the years clinical trials have led to better outcomes for people with melanoma.

You can talk to your specialist or clinical trials nurse about the protocol (the plan for the trial) then decide whether you would like to participate. The protocol includes information about the reason for the trial, who can participate, the drugs that will be given and the tests that will need to be done during the trial. The protocol ensures that researchers in different locations all perform the trial in the same way.

It is important to realise that entering a clinical trial does not guarantee that you will receive the trial drug. Half the subjects will receive either a previously used drug or an inactive tablet (placebo).

Your doctor will discuss the possible benefits and the risks of being in a clinical trial. Possible benefits include access to the newest melanoma treatments, close monitoring by the medical team and, in the long term, better understanding of how melanoma is best treated. Possible risks include side effects from new treatments that could be worse than those of the current treatments, extra visits and tests to check on your progress.

Implications of melanoma for the family

If you have been diagnosed with and treated for melanoma, this has implications for the skin cancer risk for your children. While more than 90% of melanoma is not caused by a specific known genetic mutation (a detectable abnormality in your genetic make-up), a small percentage of melanoma cases result from something inherited from your parents. If this is the case, you may have passed this mutation on to one or more of your children. Talk to your doctor about this to help decide what, if any, tests are justified.

The fact that you have had a melanoma diagnosis also suggests you are likely to have some of the common risk factors such as light-coloured skin, eyes and hair. You are likely to have passed these characteristics to some or maybe all of your children. This is a good reason to practise and encourage good sun protection from an early age. Even if the 'children' are adults, it is worth encouraging them to practise good sun protection and to talk to their doctor about your melanoma diagnosis and the implications for their own risk.

What to ask your doctor

1 What is a melanoma and how is it different from other types of skin cancer?
2 Can I have a copy of my pathology report?
3 How thick is the melanoma? Has it spread beneath my skin?
4 Has it spread to lymph nodes or other parts of my body? What tests will you do to check on this?
5 What stage is my melanoma ?
6 What treatment do you recommend and why?
7 What are the risks and possible side effects of the treatments?
8 If my lymph nodes are removed, will I get lymphoedema?
9 What is my long-term outcome (prognosis)?
10 If the melanoma has spread, is there any treatment that I can have?
11 If I need chemotherapy, can anything be done to help control the side effects?
12 How will I know if the treatment is working?
13 Are there any clinical trials of new treatments?
14 Will this new treatment be expensive?
15 Should I get a second opinion?
16 Is there someone with melanoma I can speak to?
17 Are my children at risk of getting a melanoma? Should they see a doctor ?

Further reading

Adelaide Melanoma Unit: www.rah.sa.gov.au/cancer/melanoma.php.

Australian and New Zealand Melanoma Trials Group: www.anzmtg.org/.

Cancer Council Australia: www.cancer.org.au.

Melanoma Institute of Australia: www.melanoma.org.au/.

Melanoma Patients of Australia: www.melanomapatients.org.au/.

Melanoma WA: www.melanomawa.org.au/.

Peter MacCallum Cancer Centre: www.petermac.org/.

Sydney Melanoma Unit: www.melanoma.net.au/.

Victorian Melanoma Service: victorianmelanomaservice.org/.

Western Australian Melanoma Advisory Service: www.sjog.org.au/hospitals/subiaco_hospital/
hospital_services/other_services/melanoma_advisory_service.aspx.

Chapter 11

Treatment of non-melanoma skin cancers

Victoria Snaidr, Alvin H. Chong and Peter Foley

Key messages

- Non-melanoma skin cancer (NMSC) is by far Australia's most common form of cancer, with 900 000 lesions being treated a year by 2015 at a cost in excess of $600 million.
- The vast majority of NMSCs can be treated successfully; however, in 2011 in Australia more than 500 deaths were due to NMSCs.
- Basal cell carcinoma (BCC) is the most common and least dangerous NMSC. Squamous cell carcinoma is less common but more likely to cause greater damage and, in extreme cases, death.
- Keratinocyte dysplasia, solar (or actinic) keratosis and Bowen's disease are all skin conditions that are not cancer, but that have the potential to progress into cancer.
- The majority of NMSCs are treated with surgery. For some NMSCs and keratinocyte dysplasia, other treatment options including topical cream treatment, cryotherapy using liquid nitrogen, or curettage (scraping) may also be used. In some cases radiotherapy may also be required.
- Treatment seeks to not only remove the skin cancer and any nearby cancer cells, but also to minimise other side effects, including minimising any scarring and disfigurement.
- Due to NMSCs being so common in Australia we have a lot experience in treating it. The standard of care is generally very high and the outcomes excellent.

Introduction

Non-melanoma skin cancer (NMSC) is the most common cancer in Australia, accounting for over 80% of all cancers. Two out of three Australians are diagnosed with an NMSC by the age of 70. There is a strong correlation between lifetime sun exposure, increased age and the development of NMSCs. With Australia's increasing ageing population, sunny environment and outdoor culture, the number of NMSC treatments are expected to rise to over 900 000 by 2015, placing huge economic and health care burdens on the Australian population, health care systems and government.

NMSC is the most costly cancer in Australia. Estimates show that the total treatment cost of NMSCs in 2010 was $512.3 million. This cost is projected to rise to $626.8 million in 2015.

The most common forms of NMSCs

A non-melanoma skin cancer (NMSC) describes a group of skin cancers other than melanomas. The most common NMSCs are basal cell carcinoma (BCC) and squamous cell carcinoma (SCC).

Keratinocyte dysplasia, solar (or actinic) keratosis and Bowen's disease refer to lesions that are not cancerous but may potentially be pre-cancerous. These are also linked to high levels of sun exposure.

Unlike other cancers, NMSCs are not reportable to most cancer registries in Australia. This makes calculating the incidence (number of new cases per year) of NMSCs difficult. However, it is estimated that over 767 000 NMSC lesions were treated in Australia in 2010.

Why treat NMSCs?

The goal of treatment of NMSCs is to prevent localised complications such as ulceration, bleeding and infection, and damage to underlying structures. While it is rare, preventing malignant spreading disease is also vital.

Basal cell carcinomas

Basal cell carcinoma (BCC) is the most common and least dangerous type of skin cancer. Almost 70% of skin cancers in Australia are BCCs.

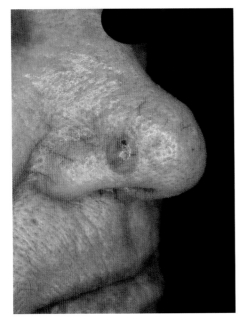

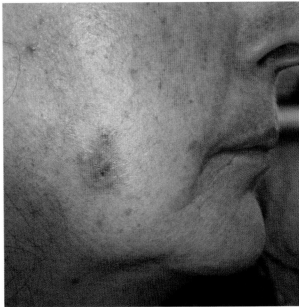

Fig. 11.1: A BCC on the nose. **Fig. 11.2:** A BCC on the cheek.

They grow slowly over months or years and only very rarely spread to distant parts of the body. Left untreated, they may ulcerate and cause damage to underlying structures. When this damage is in an area such as the eyelid or nose, it can lead to disruptions in functioning and poor cosmetic outcomes (Figs 11.1, 11.2).

There are three main different types of BCCs. The type of BCC is important to determine prognostic outcomes and direct treatment. BCC are easily treated if detected early.

Epidemiology/risk factors

Sun exposure

BCCs grow in areas chronically exposed to the sun, such as the head and neck. Living closer to the equator (e.g. northern Australia compared with southern Australia) is an independent risk factor, as is a history of working and spending a lot of time outdoors.

Age, sex

Older age increases your risk for BCC. The average age of onset is 69 years. Men are at a higher risk of developing BCCs, as are people with fair skin types (blue eyes, fair hair and freckles).

Risk factors for the development of BCCs

- Being male.
- Over age of 40.
- Personal history of cumulative sun exposure and outdoor work.
- People living closer to the equator (the highest rates of BCC are found in northern Australia).
- Sun-exposed areas of the body (head and neck, trunk).
- Fair skin.

Change

BCCs are a type of changing lesion – they grow over months to years. They are usually not painful or tender. As they grow they can ulcerate, bleed, form scabs, change or develop colour, and become tender or itchy.

Previous BCC

A family or personal history of having previous NMSCs or melanoma also places you at a higher risk of developing further BCCs.

Types of BCCs: clinical features

There are three main types of BCC, defined by their histological (microscopic) pattern of cell growth: superficial, nodular and morphoeic. 50% of all BCCs are nodular, making this the most common. Superficial BCCs are typically located on the trunk. Morphoeic BCC, although rare, is the most aggressive growth variant.

The differentiation between the three is made both clinically (how they look with the naked eye) and histologically (by examining the pattern of cells under the microscope).

Nodular BCC

A nodular BCC is the most common subtype. It is raised and slow-growing. Nodular BCCs are seldom painful or tender on palpation (pressing or touching). These lesions have a pinky-pearly translucency and a clear, well-circumscribed border. Sometimes they ulcerate and bleed (see Figs 11.3, 11.4). They are sometimes described as a 'rodent ulcer' as they are slowly invasive, like progressive rat bites.

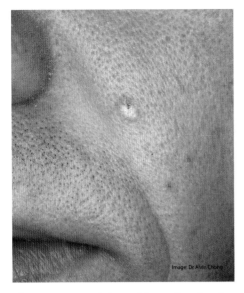

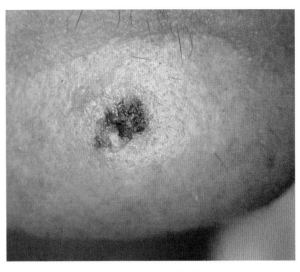

Fig. 11.3: A nodular BCC on the cheek.

Fig. 11.4: An ulcerating BCC, also known as a 'rodent ulcer'.

Superficial BCC

Superficial BCCs are more flat in appearance. They spread along the topmost (superficial) layers of the skin and are most commonly found on the trunk. They are a well-demarcated red-pink patch, slow-growing and may ulcerate or bleed (see Fig. 11.5).

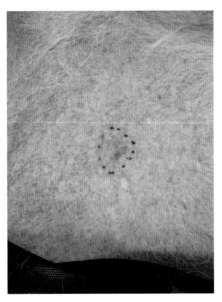

Fig. 11.5: A superficial BCC on the chest.

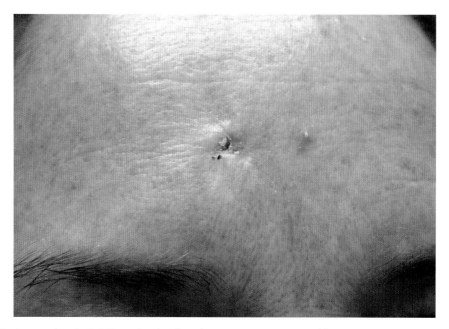

Fig. 11.6: A morphoeic BCC on the forehead presenting as a scar-like area.

Morphoeic BCC

The morphoeic subtype of BCC is not as common as the other two. These tend to be more aggressive in their growth and spread. Morphoeic BCCs can present as just a small bump but may extend deeply into the skin and surrounding structures. Often they resemble a scar (see Fig. 11.6). Due to their aggressive nature, treatment is usually with a specialist surgical procedure called Mohs' micrographic surgery, named after its pioneer, Dr Fredrick Mohs. This procedure combines surgery with on-the-spot microscopic examination of the removed specimen to ensure all of it has been removed. This procedure is discussed below, in the section on 'What about the more invasive cases?'

Diagnosis

Dermatoscope

To help make and/or confirm a diagnosis, the doctor may examine your lesion with a dermatoscope (see Fig. 9.16, p. 169). This is an instrument combining a microscope and a light source. It magnifies the structural features of your lesion, enabling the doctor to see specific characteristics for better diagnosis (see Fig. 11.7). More information on the dermatoscope is in Chapter 9, 'Early detection'.

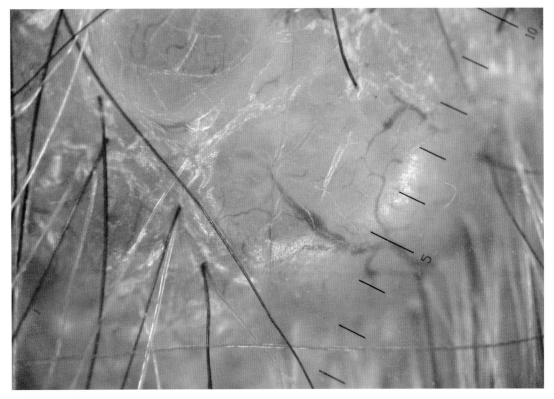

Fig. 11.7: Dermatoscopic view of a nodular BCC.

Pathology/histology

If a doctor is unsure about a lesion, they may choose to perform a preliminary biopsy to confirm the diagnosis. This involves taking a small sample of your skin for examination under a microscope.

Under the microscope, the histopathologist is able to confirm a diagnosis and identify the subtype of BCC. This helps with deciding on treatment options.

Treatment

Surgical removal or excision (with a margin of 2–3 mm) is the treatment of choice for BCCs.

For certain superficial BCCs other treatment options can be considered. These include destructive measures such as cryotherapy (the application of -196°C temperatures to 'freeze' the lesion) or curettage ('scraping' the lesion off the skin's surface). Topical immunotherapy using imiquimod (marketed under the name Aldara) cream applications can also be used. 'Topical' treatment is treatment that is applied directly on the skin, usually in the form of a cream or lotion

Key points

- BCCs are *changing* skin cancer lesions.
- Biopsies are performed to establish pre-treatment diagnosis.
- Dermatoscopic examination enhances diagnosis.
- Sun exposure, age and being male increase your risk of BCCs.
- Having a prior history of BCC increases your risk of developing another.

that destroys sun-damaged cells via the body's own inflammatory process. Radiation treatment is an option for certain BCCs. More detail on treatments is given later in the chapter.

Prognosis

With complete removal, the prognosis of BCC is excellent. Incomplete removal has a 30% recurrence rate. Recurrence is when the disease comes back.

Follow-up

Having been diagnosed with one BCC increases your risk of developing another in the future. This risk is the reason why you have regular reviews by your doctor, especially with any concerning or changing lesions.

Squamous cell carcinomas

Squamous cell carcinomas (SCCs) are less common, but potentially more dangerous than BCCs. They typically grow quickly (over weeks to months). If not treated promptly, they have a greater potential to spread past their boundaries and to other parts of the body.

Most SCCs develop from lesions called solar keratoses or actinic keratoses (SKs, AKs). SKs are collections of sun-damaged skin cells. They present as a thickened, scaly red lesion, which may bleed or ulcerate and may also be sore or tender. These lesions commonly develop in the sun-exposed areas of the body such as the hands, forearms, head and neck.

Epidemiology and risk factors

Estimates indicate ~30% of all skin cancers in Australia are SCCs. Similarly to BCCs, they are more common in males, in people over the age of 40, and with high levels of cumulative sun exposure (e.g. outdoor workers, people living closer to the equator – northern Australia).

In men, SCCs most commonly occur in the head and neck areas. In women, they commonly develop along the arms.

Clinical features

SCCs present as pink papules or nodules (raised swellings) with an overlying hyperkeratosis (scaly patch). They grow in size over a matter of weeks to months, and as they grow can become painful and tender. They may also ulcerate or bleed (Fig. 11.8).

On occasion (~1 in 100), SCCs can grow outside their boundaries (locally aggressive) and/or spread to local lymph nodes or other parts of the body (metastasise). The likelihood of this happening increases in people whose immunity is suppressed (e.g. organ transplant patients, patients with autoimmune conditions who are on long-term immune-suppressive medications). Other characteristics of SCCs which are aggressive include location on certain parts of the body such as lips, scalp and ears, rapidly growing tumours, deeply invasive or thick tumours, tumours which invade nerves, and tumours which show poor differentiation when analysed under the microscope.

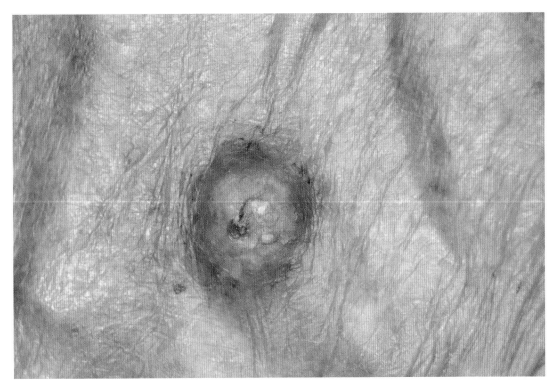

Fig. 11.8: An SCC on the hand.

Diagnosis

Differentiating SCCs from other scaly lesions due to sun damage, such as Bowen's disease (SCC in situ) or solar keratoses can be difficult (Figs 11.9–11.13). A preliminary biopsy may be needed to help your doctor confirm the diagnosis before deciding on further management.

Treatment options

Surgical removal or excision is the treatment of choice for SCCs. Removing a lesion with clear margins reduces the chance of it recurring (returning). Incomplete removal of an SCC creates a 50% chance of recurrence. Some SCCs require further treatment with radiotherapy, particularly if they involve nerves.

Prognosis

With complete excision, SCC generally have good prognoses. Poor outcomes are more common in deeper lesions, lesions involving nerves, those that have spread past their boundaries or those located on the scalp, ear and the edge of the lip.

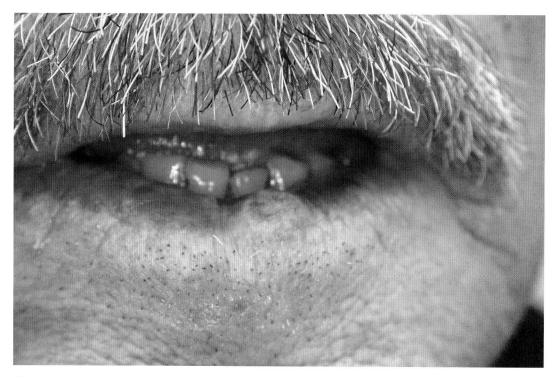

Fig. 11.9: An SCC on the lip.

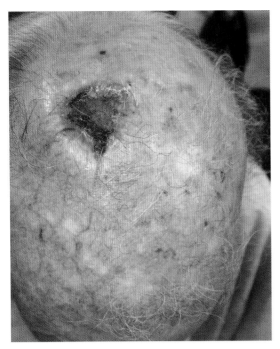

Fig. 11.10: An SCC on the scalp.

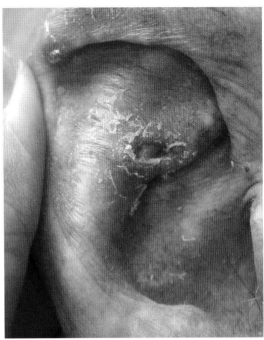

Fig. 11.11: An SCC on the ear.

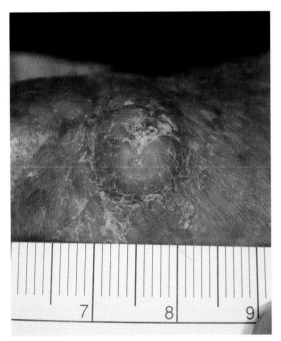

Fig. 11.12: An SCC on the hand.

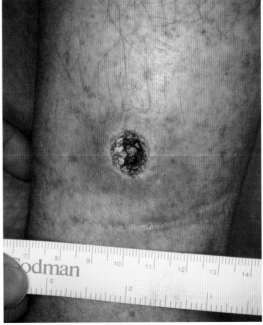

Fig. 11.13: An SCC on the lower leg.

Follow-up

Once you have been diagnosed with an SCC, you are at a higher risk of developing another, either at the same site or in a different location. Being familiar with your skin and having regular annual skin checks is therefore vital for good skin health.

Keratoacanthomas

Keratoacanthomas are thought to be a type of well-differentiated SCC (Fig. 11.14). They tend to grow quickly over a few months and can reach diameters of 2 cm. Keratoacanthomas differ from typical SCCs in that they can regress (shrink and disappear) over a span of time. The current recommendation is for complete excision given the concern for SCC.

Other types of premalignant skin lesions

Keratocyte dysplasia

Keratocyte dysplasias also arise from sun-damaged skin cells. The term 'keratocyte dysplasia' essentially means an abnormal thickening and overgrowth of the topmost layer of the skin. These lesions are not invasive cancers, but have the potential to become cancerous.

Solar/actinic keratoses

Solar keratoses (SK), also known as actinic keratoses, arise from areas of sun damage. They appear as a patch of flat or thickened skin, which can be either skin-coloured or red, and rough to touch (Fig. 11.15). An associated itching or burning sensation may be present. Occasionally they may grow a cutaneous horn. Typically, they are not tender.

There is a small risk of an SK developing into an SCC. This is reported as approximately one in 1000 per year. There should be concern of transformation (becoming an SCC) in any changing lesion over time, e.g. tenderness, growth, increased thickness of lesion.

A past history of significant sun exposure coupled with a fair skin type is a common predisposing factor in developing SKs. If you have been diagnosed with an SK, regular skin examination is recommended as you are at an increased risk of developing other NMSCs.

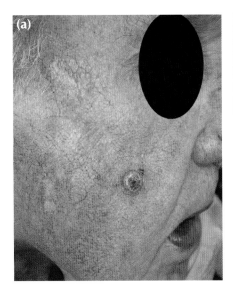

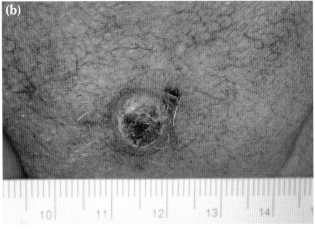

Fig. 11.14: (a) A keratoacanthoma on the cheek.
(b) Close-up of a keratoacanthoma.

SCC in situ (Bowen's disease)

Bowen's disease has a flat, reddened, scaly, patchy appearance, and is most commonly asymptomatic (Figs 11.16, 11.17). It is termed an SCC in situ – it is a precursor to SCC but is confined to the epidermis (the outermost layer of the skin). The risk of SCC in situ progressing to invasive SCC is approximately 5–10% per year. Lesions are treated to ensure complete removal and reduce their risk for progressing to SCC.

Treatment options include surgical removal and topical creams. These are discussed later.

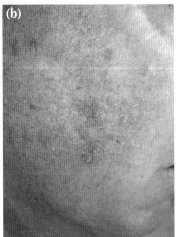

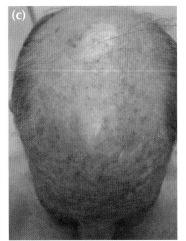

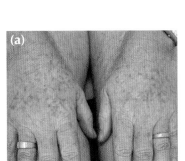

Fig. 11.15: (a) SKs on the hands, (b) cheeks and (c) scalp.

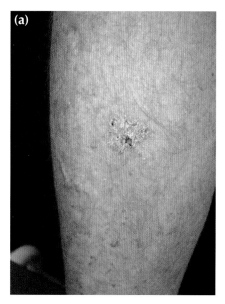
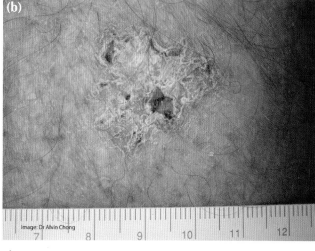

Fig. 11.16: (a) SCC in situ on the leg. (b) A close-up view.

Common ways to treat NMSCs and keratinocyte dysplasia

Invasive NMSCs (SCCs, nodular and morphoeic BCCs) are mainly treated by surgical excision. Superficial BCCs and keratinocyte dysplasia may be treated by other means such as destructive modalities, topical therapies and surgical excision. 'Destructive modalities' are treatments that

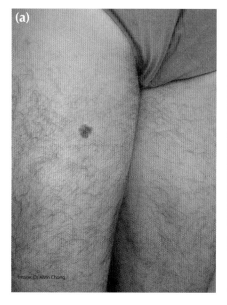
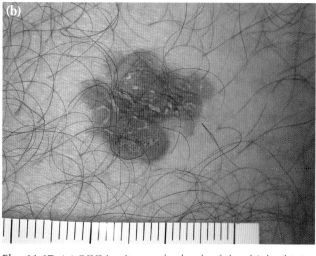

Fig. 11.17: (a) SCC in situ on the back of the thigh. (b) A close-up view.

physically change or destroy the skin and the lesion, i.e. cutting, scraping or freezing. These are different from 'topical modalities', which achieve the change using chemical reactions with the skin and the lesion.

Topical therapies

Topical therapies are applied to the surface of the skin and are commonly creams and lotions, with varying modes of action. All the topical therapies listed below destroy sun-damaged and abnormal cells in preference to normal cells.

It is recommended that topical therapies should always be applied to clean dry skin, using either a metal applicator or with gloves, and as directed by your doctor. All these modalities can irritate normal undamaged skin so washing your hands well after use and avoiding touching your eyes or eyelids is important to avoid irritation or damage to healthy skin.

It is important to avoid the sun during treatment by any of the listed therapies.

The duration of treatment varies between products. An awareness of what to expect is important. This avoids disappointments with the product and gives you an idea of when to seek help in preventing adverse effects and long-term complications.

Your doctor may choose to confirm the diagnosis of your lesion with a skin biopsy before starting any treatment. This is usually either a shave or a punch biopsy

5% 5-fluorouracil cream

In Australia 5% 5-fluorouracil cream (marketed as Efudix) is mainly used to treat SKs and Bowen's disease. Overseas it is sometimes used to treat superficial BCCs. 5-fluorouracil is a cream that is applied once or twice daily for several weeks. The duration and frequency of treatment depends on the type and site of lesion being treated.

Typical side effects include a stinging or burning sensation, redness, irritation, scaling, blistering, sores and crusts.

5-fluorouracil can be considered a form of chemotherapy applied to the skin; it destroys sun-damaged cells by affecting their ability to reproduce. It interrupts the cell-cycle and induces cell death by blocking an important step in the skin cell's replication cycle. It has been described as topical chemotherapy for the skin.

Sun-damaged cells have a tendency to replicate faster, and less efficiently. They absorb and incorporate 5-fluorouracil faster than the surrounding healthy cells; this is how it destroys abnormal cells, with less chance of harming healthy cells.

Cure rates

Information on efficacy rates for the treatment of SKs and Bowen's disease are limited.

Table 11.1: 5% 5-fluorouracil cream – how to apply

Lesion	Application method	Notes
SK	Once to twice daily for 2–4 weeks on the head and neck	The area of treatment should not exceed 500 cm^2 (approx. 23 × 23 cm)
Bowen's disease	Once to twice daily for 4–8 weeks	Larger areas should be treated a section at a time
		Consider treating in winter or cooler seasons to avoid worsening or exaggeration of side effects by the sun
		Not to be used by women who are breastfeeding or pregnant

3% Diclofenac sodium in 2.5% hyaluronan gel

3% Diclofenac sodium gel (marketed as Solaraze) is approved by the TGA in Australia for the treatment of solar keratosis.

It is a gel containing a non-steroidal anti-inflammatory component, similar to that used in some arthritis medications. It inhibits several enzymes within cells and destroys sun-damaged skin cells by decreasing new blood vessel formation within the 'tumour', reducing cell turnover and triggering cell death. Treatment typically lasts for 30–90 days. It is generally well tolerated, though side effects can include itching, redness, irritation, rash, dryness, scaling or peeling.

Table 11.2: 3% Diclofenac sodium gel – how to apply

Lesion	TGA approved application method	Notes
SK	Twice daily for 90 days total	The recommended application for 90 days results in 50% complete clearance
		In more hypertrophic (thicker) or resistant lesions, may be used in combination with cryotherapy

Imiquimod 5% cream

Imiquimod 5% cream (marketed as Aldara) has been approved by the TGA in Australia for the treatment of superficial BCCs and SKs.

It stimulates the body's natural immune response to target and destroy abnormal, sun-damaged cells by binding to toll-like receptor 7, which is important in recognition of viral infections, on immune cells. Imiquimod stimulates several of the body's immune cells to produce various proteins, including interferon, that fight the cancerous cells.

5% imiquimod cream can also be used for Bowen's disease. There is limited data on imiquimod's efficacy in nodular BCCs. The TGA has not approved the use of 5% imiquimod for use in those lesions.

Table 11.3: Imiquimod 5% cream – how to apply

Lesion	TGA approved application method	Notes
Superficial BCCs	Once daily 5× per week (e.g. Monday–Friday) for 6 weeks total	Apply cream to tumour plus margin of 5 mm Review efficacy of treatment at 2–3 months
Solar keratoses	Once daily 3× per week (e.g Monday, Wednesday, Friday) up to 16 weeks total	In practice, most clinicians advise: 2–3× per week for 2–4 weeks Cycle may be repeated after a month for increased efficacy Rest periods are necessary if the inflammatory reaction becomes excessive +/– low-dose topical steroid
Nodular BCCs	Not approved	*May* be beneficial as an adjunct to curettage and electrodesiccation (once daily × 4 weeks) *May* be considered for use if other treatment options are contraindicated Should not be used for morphoeic, infiltrating or micronodular subtypes of BCCs
SCC in situ (Bowen's disease)	Not approved	In practice, most clinicians advise: Once daily 3–4× per week for 4–6 weeks in total Review during treatment may be necessary due to excessive inflammatory response in some patients

Ingenol mebutate 0.015%, 0.05%

Ingenol mebutate (marketed as Picato) is a topical treatment derived from the plant *Euphorbia peplus*. It works by inducing cell death via necrosis and inflammation. Ingenol mebutate's benefit is a reduced duration of therapy. Depending on the site treated, only two or three days of treatment are needed.

For the treatment of SKs on the face and scalp, ingenol mebutate 0.015% gel (lower strength) is used on the affected area once daily for three consecutive days. For SKs on the trunk and limbs, ingenol mebutate 0.05% gel (higher strength) is applied once daily for two consecutive days. The complete clearance of SKs was reported as 42.2% on the face and scalp and 34.1% on the trunk and limbs.

There may be significant local inflammatory skin reactions which peak between days 3 and 8, declining to baseline levels by day 29. Unlike other topical treatments, sun protection is not required during therapy with this agent.

Table 11.4: Ingenol mebutate – how to apply

Lesion	TGA approved application method	Notes
SK – face and scalp	Ingenol mebutate 0.015% Once daily for 3 days total	The lower-strength 0.015% is used for face and scalp Higher-strength 0.05% for trunk and extremities Inflammation may occur for up to a week following treatment
SK – trunk and extremities	Ingenol mebutate 0.05% Once daily for 2 days total	

Salicylic acid

Salicylic acid is applied to the skin in a cream or ointment base and is effective in treating thickened, scaling skin lesions. It penetrates and dissolves the thickened top layers of the skin (the stratum corneum), as often seen in SCCs and SKs.

How to apply

5–10% salicyclic acid cream can be applied once daily as needed to keep lesions flat.

Photodynamic therapy (PDT)

In this form of treatment, light (in the form of long-wave visible or infrared radiation) is directed onto an area of the body that has been sensitised with a light-sensitising cream. This cream is applied to the skin and absorbed into damaged cells where it undergoes a chemical change and once activated by light, causes their destruction. It is reserved for use in specialist dermatology clinics as it requires specialist training and equipment.

PDT can be used to treat a variety of skin lesions including SKs, superficial BCCs and Bowen's disease. The recurrence rate is higher in nodular BCCs. PDT is not recommended for the treatment of SCCs, given high recurrence rates. Cosmetically, PDT generally provides good results with minimal scarring.

Table 11.5: Photodynamic therapy – how to apply

Lesion	Regime	Notes
SK	Single session with review at 3 months	A second session may be necessary if lesion persists Cream applied to prepared treatment field, left under a dressing for 3 hours then removed, followed by illumination with intense light or laser
Superficial BCC, Bowen's disease	2 sessions, one week apart	

Destructive modalities

Cryotherapy

Cryotherapy refers to the use of low temperatures to treat skin tumours. It involves directing liquid nitrogen (LiqN$_2$) on to a lesion with either a cotton tip applicator or a spray nozzle. It is used for the treatment of SKs, small superficial BCCs and SCCs in situ. A variety of benign skin lesions that are not in the skin cancer spectrum are also treated with cryotherapy. These include seborrhoeic keratoses, viral warts, solar lentigo, porokeratosis, myxoid cysts and molluscum contagiosum in adults. Other uses of cryotherapy include skin tags (although snip excision may be preferred), keloid scars (combined with intralesional steroids) and some vascular lesions. However, for vascular lesions diathermy and laser are usually considered better options.

The 'double-freeze thaw' method is effective in the treatment of BCCs, while generally only a single freeze is required for SKs. The double-freeze thaw method involves two cycles (up to 15 seconds long) of liquid nitrogen applied to the lesions.

Cryotherapy works via two mechanisms. First, it destroys the damaged tissue by directly exposing it to -196°C. Second, it stimulates a local inflammatory reaction which encourages the body's own natural defences to destroy the affected tissue.

Side effects or complications of cryotherapy can be divided into immediate, short-term and long-term. Immediate effects include local pain, headache (when spots on the head are treated), fainting, swelling, redness and (rarely) air within the skin (soft tissue insufflation). Short-term effects include blister formation (24–48 hours), crusting, bleeding, pain, infection, delayed healing and excessive granulation tissue formation (overexuberant wound healing similar to what is seen with an ingrown toenail). Potential long-term effects include disturbances of skin colour (lighter or darker), scarring, nerve damage, hair loss and notching of free margins such as ear, lip border and eyelid (ectropion). There may be recurrence of lesions.

In general, cryotherapy is a simple, quick, convenient, low-cost, well-tolerated technique that does not require anaesthesia and gives a reasonable cosmetic outcome.

How to apply
2 × 15 second applications to the lesion, allowing to thaw between cycles.

Curettage
Curettage is a technique of tissue destruction that removes, by scraping or scooping, predominantly superficial (epidermal) skin lesions with a sharp, spoon-like instrument (a circular scalpel). The sun-damaged cells are more friable (easily separated) and are easily removed with a 'scraping' motion.

It is useful in treating superficial BCCs, SCCs in situ and other lesions which extend to only the surface layers of the skin. A range of benign skin lesions may also be treated with this technique, including seborrhoeic keratoses, molluscum contagiosum, pyogenic granuloma, milia, warts and sebaceous hyperplasia.

Often, diathermy (applying heat to close bleeding capillaries) is used following curettage to achieve haemostasis (stop the bleeding) and to further destroy remaining cancerous cells.

Short-term side effects include pain, bleeding, delayed wound healing, itch and infection, while medium- to long-term complications include scarring, pigment disturbance and recurrence.

Biopsies and excisions

Biopsies

A biopsy is a procedure where a small sample of skin is taken for microscopic examination to confirm the diagnosis of a skin cancer. Common techniques are the punch biopsy and the shave biopsy.

Punch biopsies

A punch biopsy uses a sharp utensil to remove a cylindrical core of skin sample through all layers of the skin, at a diameter of 2–4 mm. This type of biopsy is important when information regarding the depth of your lesion is needed.

Depending on its size, a punch biopsy will either be left to heal on its own or the doctor may close the defect with a suture (stitch).

Shave biopsies

A shave biopsy takes only the top few layers of the skin. It is useful in lesions where sun-damaged cells are located in only the superficial layers of your skin, eg superficial BCCs and Bowen's disease.

Shave biopsies tend leave small flat scars. This is because only the top surface of the skin is removed. Hypopigmented (pale) scars can still occur in patients with olive or darker skin.

Excisions

An excision is the surgical removal (cutting out) of a lesion. The choice to remove a lesion surgically is based on microscopic diagnosis, location (on the body or head), size of the lesion, ease of procedure and patient preference.

Surgical excisions range from simple procedures such as excision and primary side-to-side closure, to more complex excisions requiring flap-repairs and skin grafts. Depending on the size, site and closure options, surgical excisions can be relatively quick (no more than a few minutes) to a half-day commitment. They provide excellent cure rates by removing affected tissues in their entirety.

Treatment of more invasive cases

Although it's rare, NMSCs, particularly SCCs, can potentially spread past their local boundaries (locally advanced spread) and invade other parts of the body (metastatic spread).

In these situations, the use of radiotherapy, chemotherapy or a more specialist surgical technique (Mohs micrographic surgery) can be considered.

Radiotherapy

Radiotherapy uses X-rays to destroy sun-damaged cells of the skin. It is used to treat BCCs or SCCs that have either spread beyond treatment by simple measures, or in situations where other methods may not be appropriate.

The area of the skin is marked and exposed to high-frequency X-rays, which destroy the cells by damaging the DNA within them. A protective shield is placed over healthy skin surrounding the tumour. The X-rays affect normal cells surrounding the area of sun-damaged skin lesion, but healthy cells have a better ability to repair themselves than sun-damaged tumour cells.

Radiotherapy is delivered at specialised centres. Each treatment (a 'fraction') does not take longer than a few minutes. A treatment regime varies from a few treatment sessions per week to daily treatments for several weeks. The duration and regime of treatment depends on the size, type and position of your skin cancer, and will be decided by your specialist.

Damaged skin cells slowly accumulate radiation to a level from which they cannot recover or repair themselves, and so undergo cell death. Normal cells exposed to X-rays should be able to repair themselves before the next treatment.

In some cases, radiotherapy is used in addition to surgery (Fig. 11.18). This may be prior to surgery (to reduce the size of a lesion for a better surgical outcome) or after surgery (to ensure all damaged cells have been treated, thereby reducing the risk of the cancer recurring).

Utilising radiotherapy

- When lesions cover a large area of the body.
- When lesions are located in an area where it is difficult to perform surgery.
- Where post-surgical repair may be poor and scarring may occur.
- In people who do not want surgery.
- In people who are not fit for surgery.

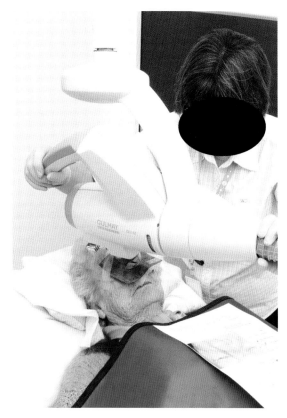

Fig. 11.18: Radiotherapy being applied to the nose.

Side effects

It is usual for the area exposed to radiation to turn red, which may become permanent, throughout the duration of treatment. The area may also develop crusting or weeping. This should subside a short time after the radiation treatment has been completed.

Should the ooze or crust be excessive, then bathing with cooled salty water for a few minutes followed by application of a topical dressing (Vaseline, antibiotic or antiseptic cream) twice daily is recommended.

The treated area should always be protected against sun, wind or trauma (injury).

Prognosis

Radiotherapy has a high cure rate. Recurrence is rare, but can manifest as a second cancer which develops in the same site. A radiation scar – often lighter in colour than the surrounding skin and waxy in appearance – may develop, as can prominent blood vessels on the surface of the skin, leaving an area of permanent redness.

Vismodegib (Hedgehog inhibitors)

Vismodegib (marketed as Erivedge, in capsule form) is a relatively new, non-surgical treatment of invasive NMSCs. It was approved in 2013 by the TGA as treatment for the rare cases of metastatic BCC, or for locally advanced BCCs where surgery and/or radiation therapy are not appropriate.

It works by stopping or inhibiting a signal within the cell, which is important for its replication. This particular signal (the Hedgehog pathway) is amplified in sun-damaged cells, which results in their rapid growth into a tumorous lesion. When this signal is arrested, the damaged cells are unable to replicate. This prevents further expansion and growth of the tumour.

Vismodegib is taken as a 150 mg capsule daily until the tumour resolves. Similar to radiotherapy, vismodegib can be used to shrink the tumour before surgery.

Recent clinical trials show an overall response rate of 30–43% in non-operable BCCs.

Possible side effects include muscle spasms (cramps), alopecia (hair loss) and taste disturbance.

Given promising results in these types of skin cancers, vismodegib is currently undergoing clinical trials for use in other cancers such as stomach cancer, pancreatic cancer, prostate cancer and lung cancer.

Mohs micrographic surgery

Mohs micrographic surgery is a specialised surgery which is used where a skin cancer has spread beyond its visible clinical margins. This type of surgery is performed by dermatologists who have been specially trained in micrographic surgery. It takes longer than a routine excision; it may take several hours, or even half a day. The Mohs surgeon will excise your lesion and while you wait in the recovery room, process the removed tissue onto slides for examination under a microscope. The surgeon will take particular care with each boundary of the excised lesion, to ensure that the entire area of sun-damaged cells has been removed.

With a standard skin excision the removed tissue is sliced like a loaf of bread and the edges of several slices are examined to determine if all the tumour is 'out', with the Mohs technique the excision specimen is peeled like an orange so that all the edge may be examined.

If there is any residual cancer, another stage of surgery is carried out and the whole process is repeated until no cancer cells remain in any removed skin tissue. As the area excised is carefully mapped, the additional stage of surgery only removes involved additional skin. Only after all the cancer has been removed does the surgeon plan to close the wound.

It is important to know that, although your naked eye may see only a small lesion, the spread of sun-damaged or affected cells may spread beyond the visible boundaries. This spread of damaged cells can only be determined with the microscopic examination of the cells which have been removed. As a result, on occasion a much larger area of skin needs to be removed (in comparison to the size of the original visible lesion). Your Mohs surgeon needs special surgical skills to ensure good cosmetic results, as most wound defects require skin grafts or flap-repairs to close the large wound.

Risks and complications

As with any surgical procedure, the most common side effects include bleeding, bruising, swelling, pain and infection.

Long-term complications include incomplete removal of the tumour, and scarring.

Deciding which treatment to apply

There is often more than one way to treat an NMSC (Fig. 11.19). Treatment choice is not only dependent on diagnosis, but takes into account factors such as:

1   type of lesion – the histological diagnosis of a lesion dictates the choice of therapy for treatment. For example, lesions such as SCCs are always recommended for surgical removal, but some lesions such as Bowen's and superficial BCCs have more options for removal, e.g. topical applications like creams and lotions or destructive or surgical removal;

2   size – small simple lesions are easily treated with local surgery or topical creams. Larger lesions may need concurrent treatment with chemotherapy or radiotherapy;

3   anatomical location – some areas are very difficult to treat surgically (e.g. nasal folds, ears) and other areas such as the lower limbs have poorer healing ability. In such cases, radiotherapy or topical treatment may be more appropriate;

4   number of lesions – the number of lesions you have as well as the size of the area they cover influences the type of treatment which would adequately treat your NMSCs. For example, multiple NMSCs covering a large area of your back may be better treated with topical therapy whereas a small, solitary lesion may be best treated with surgical removal;

5   patient request/tolerance – your doctor should always discuss all possible options available to adequately treat your skin cancer. You may have had a particularly bad or good experience with one type of therapy; if so, it is important to inform your treating doctor as there may be a an alternative possibility should you not tolerate or prefer one particular treatment type.

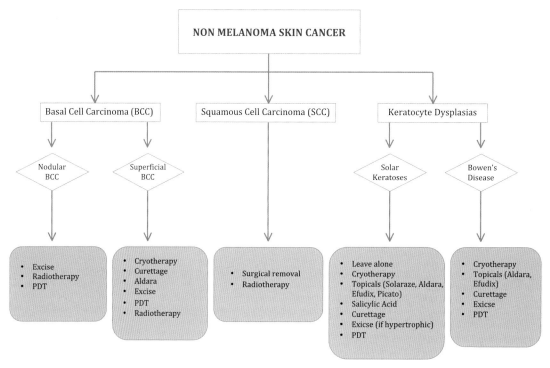

Fig. 11.19: Treatment options for NMSCs.

Cosmetic effects of treatment options

It is important to have an understanding of what your skin will look like (i.e. the cosmetic effect) during and following different therapies. Often, with many of the topical therapies, your skin may look much worse before it improves. An understanding of the common reactions to these therapies is important to prevent disappointment in the product and to help you know when to seek medical advice for adverse reactions.

Topical therapies

5% 5-fluorouracil cream

Sun-damaged areas of skin treated with 5-fluorouracil undergo destruction through a severe inflammatory process. Within a week or two, the areas treated with 5-fluorouracil will turn red, become inflamed and may begin to crust. This reaction is typical and is necessary for the cream to be able to destroy the sun-damaged cells. This reaction can be quite unsightly (Figs 11.20, 11.21), so it is important to plan your treatment to avoid coinciding with any important social

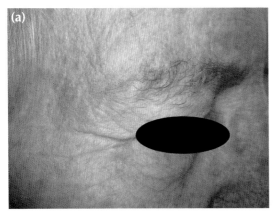 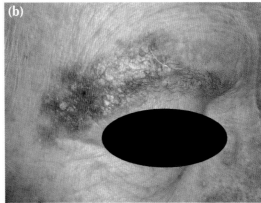

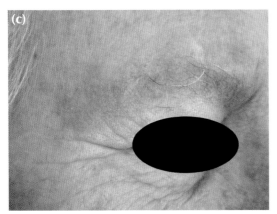

Fig. 11.20: A typical pattern of the cosmetic effect of 5-fluorouracil therapy. (a) Before, (b) during and (c) after therapy.

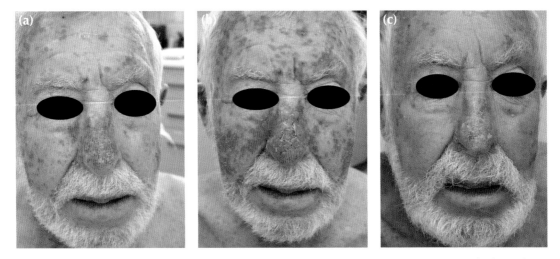

Fig. 11.21: A severe reaction to 5-fluorouracil therapy. The cosmetic appearance (a) before, (b) during and (c) after therapy.

events (weddings etc.). On occasion, a topical cortisone cream may be prescribed to dampen the degree of inflammation.

Once crusts form they can be covered with Vaseline or gently soaked off with a warm water bath.

They should not be covered with gauze or bandages, unless instructed by your doctor.

Make-up can cause stinging and further irritation.

It is very important to stay out of the sun during treatment with 5-fluorouracil.

Complications can occur. Most of these includes excessive inflammatory reactions, infection and increased scaling, all of which can lead to scarring and areas of hypopigmentation (decreased skin colour).

3% Diclofenac sodium in 2.5% hyaluronan gel

Diclofenac gel is generally well tolerated. It may cause local irritation of the skin, resulting in redness, itch, dryness, scaling or peeling of the area while undergoing treatment (Fig. 11.22).

Imiquimod 5% cream

Imiquimod 5% cream's efficacy relies on an inflammatory process to destroy sun-damaged cells. As such, local redness and irritation is a common and important process.

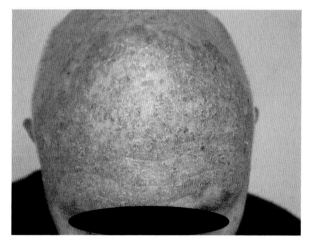
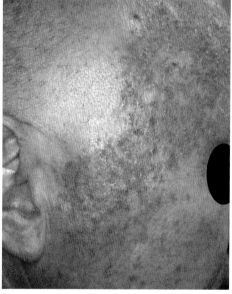

Fig. 11.22: A severe reaction to 3% Diclofenac gel.

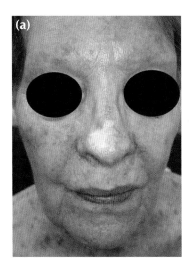

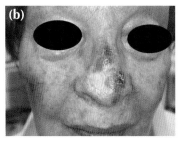

Fig. 11.23: A typical reaction to 5% imiquimod cream when used to treat facial actinic keratoses. (a) Before, (b) during and (c) after treatment.

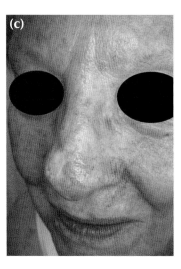

In a large clinical trial examining the effectiveness and safety of imiquimod, more than 50% of people experienced side effects, which ranged from itching and burning, to redness, flaking/scaling, swelling, ulcerations and crusting/scabbing (Figs 11.23–11.26).

Ingenol mebutate 0.015%, 0.05%

The inflammatory response after application of ingenol mebutate typically occurs after the first day; peak reactions, in terms of skin redness, flaking/scaling and crusting, intensify within a

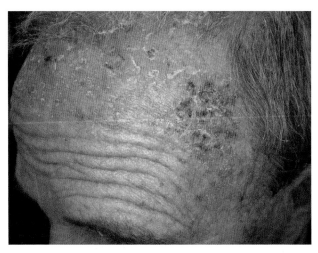

Fig. 11.24: Treating AK with 5% imiquimod cream.

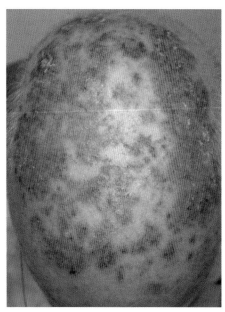

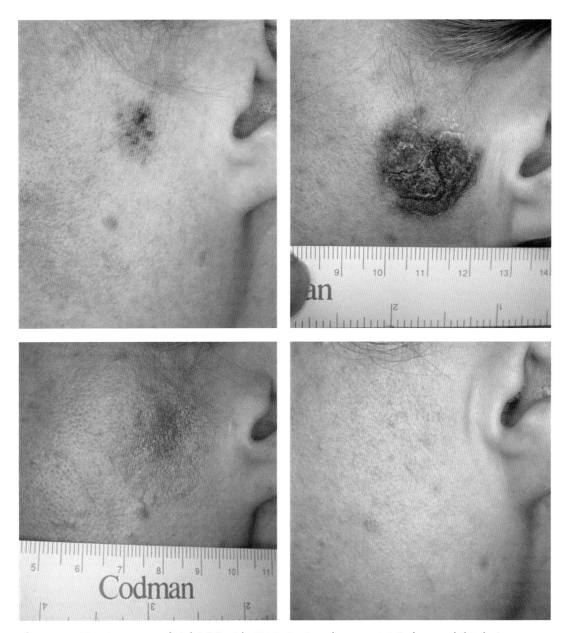

Fig. 11.25: Treating a superficial BCC with 5% imiquimod cream. (a) Before and (b) during treatment. (c) Four weeks after treatment. (d) Six months after treatment.

week of treatment. Resolution of effects typically occurs from two weeks (face and scalp) to four weeks (trunk, extremities).

Common adverse effects at the site of application include erosion, redness, swelling, scabbing, itch, pain, ulceration, irritation and peeling (Fig. 11.27).

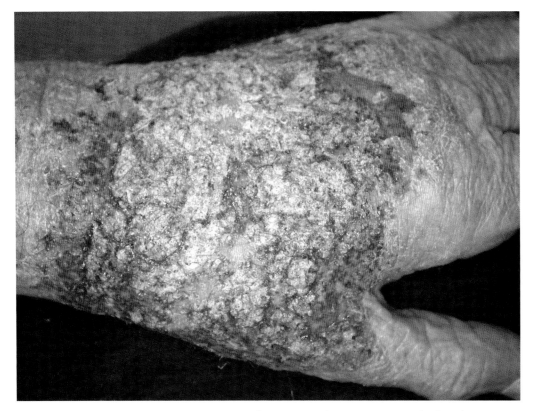

Fig. 11.26: A severe reaction to 5% imiquimod cream used to treat AKs on the hand.

Salicylic acid

Salicylic acid is generally well tolerated with minimal side effects, although mild irritation occurs on occasion.

Destructive modalities

Cryotherapy

Following cryotherapy, a blister will typically form within a few hours. Within a few days, the blister dries and a scab forms. The scab will fall off in days to weeks, depending on the body area:

- face, 5–10 days;
- hands, 1–2 weeks;
- legs, 2–4 weeks.

Once a scab forms, the application of Vaseline or other occlusive dressing helps to avoid scab-picking and reduce scar formation.

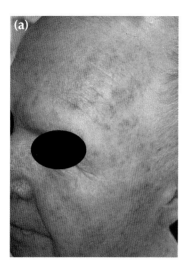

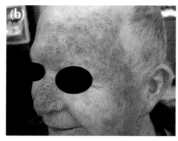

Fig. 11.27: Treating AKs with ingenol mebutate 0.015% cream. (a) Before, (b) during and (c) after treatment.

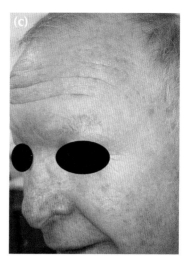

Complications occasionally occur. These may include infection, blistering, swelling, scarring and hypopigmentation.

Occasionally, cryotherapy needs to be repeated some weeks later to clear the lesion. Lesions may recur with time.

Curettage

Curettage leaves an open wound which heals through regeneration of new tissue. A scab will form within the first week. This procedure will result in some degree of scarring. Lesions may recur, requiring further treatment.

The main complications apart from bleeding include excessive scabbing, infection and increased scarring.

Surgical excisions: what to expect

Excisions will always result in some degree of scarring. The size, character and appearance of the scars depends on a multitude of factors, ranging from size of the lesions to be excised, their location on the body and the degree of success in minimising complications such as bleeding, infection and excessive tension on the healing wound.

Classically, a lesion (with a margin of apparently uninvolved skin) is removed in the shape of an ellipse. The edges of the wound are then brought together and held in place with sutures (primary closure). The length of the resulting scar is three times the diameter of the original lesion. This enables appropriate wound closure to achieve the best cosmetic results.

Some lesions can't be removed with a simple elliptical excision. Where a lesion is located in a difficult area or is too large to remove with a simple ellipse, your doctor may perform a flap-repair or a skin graft. Another option is to allow the skin to heal on its own via a process known as secondary intension wound healing or granulation repair.

Elliptical excision
As shown in Figs 11.28 and 11.29, the lesion is removed along a known crease in the facial contour. Note that the length of the excision is significantly longer than the diameter of the lesion itself. The process achieves excellent cosmetic results.

Flap repair
In this process, the lesion is removed and an adjacent area of skin is loosened and moved/rotated to cover the wound defect left by the original lesion (Figs 11.30, 11.31).

Skin graft
Occasionally, when a lesion is removed which covers a larger area or is in a location where surrounding skin is not in abundant supply, closure of the wound is achieved with a skin graft

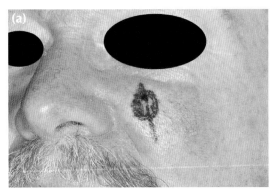

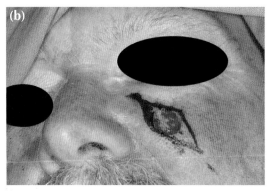

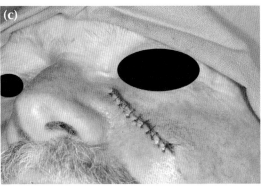

Fig. 11.28: A BCC on the cheek, removed surgically with an elliptical excision.

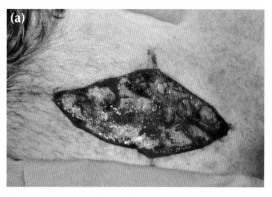

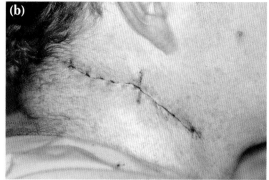

Fig. 11.29: An elliptical excision on the neck.

(Fig. 11.32). A small section of skin is removed from another area of the body (commonly the thigh, neck, behind or in front of the ear), laid over the open defect and sutured into place. The donor site that the skin graft is taken from may be left to heal by secondary intention or may be sutured (stitched).

Healing by granulation/second intention

This method of allowing the wound to heal without surgical intervention is used infrequently. It is sometimes necessary in certain areas such as the inner ear and temples. These types of open wounds take three to four weeks to heal, leave hypopigmented scars and can cause contractions.

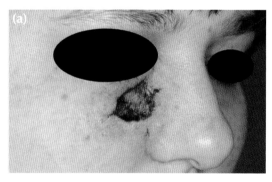

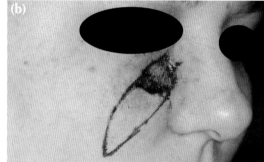

Fig. 11.30: An island pedicle flap.

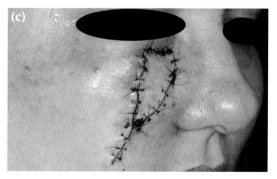

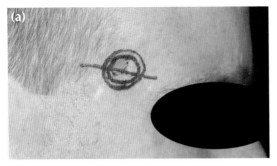

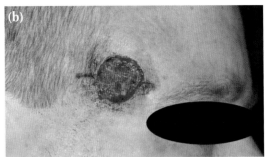

Fig. 11.31: A transposition flap.

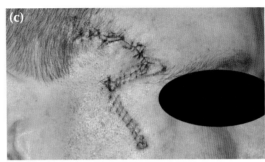

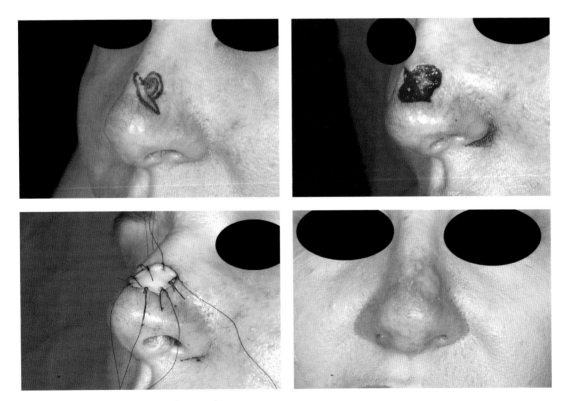

Fig. 11.32: A full-thickness skin graft.

How to manage long-lasting scars

Scars are inevitable following a skin biopsy or excision. They form as a result of the skin's natural healing process following injury, to replace the skin tissue which has been damaged or removed.

How scars form

The process of scar formation involves three phases.

The inflammatory phase (days 1–3)

The aim of this initial phase is to stop the wound from bleeding. During this phase, your body's inflammatory process is targeted to the area of the wound. It deposits cells from within the blood to form a scab made of both blood and skin cells. Other inflammatory cells from the blood arrive to remove dead tissue cells and destroy any bacteria.

The proliferative stage (days 4–21)

This is the phase when new skin tissue is created to replace the scab that formed in the inflammatory stage. New skin cells are deposited and collagen is laid down to secure the new tissue in place. Collagen adds strength and elasticity to the skin. This new tissue is called granulation tissue and is composed of lots of blood cells and new skin cells. It has a lumpy appearance and can look quite pink or red.

Healthy skin cells within the upper layer of the skin around the wound rearrange themselves to re-establish the integrity of the skin. They loosen their attachments to each other, migrate across the wound surface and come together to close the skin.

The remodelling phase (days 21–year 1)

This phase involves the maturation of the wound. The formation of granulation tissue is stopped and the excess cells and tissues which are not needed are removed. If the excess cells of granulation tissue are not removed and degraded by this process, a thickened scar often results.

The remaining cells mature into a more organised cell structure within the collagen meshwork which was laid down in the previous stage. The organisation of this collagen is never as exact as the original structure and will always look different from the original skin.

The final stage of scar formation involves scar contraction, caused by the contraction of small muscles cells within the collagen fibres in scar tissue. It is important in reducing the surface area of the scar.

Risk factors for scarring

Most scars tend to fade over time, however, long-lasting scars may occur in areas of the body under high tension (e.g. trunk, feet, shoulder) and in younger, darker-skinned people. Additional influences include chronic disease (e.g. poor circulation, diabetes, cancer, coronary artery disease, renal failure), poor lifestyle choices (smoking, alcohol, poor nutrition) and genetics.

The main factors that influence scarring and healing are:

1   age – increased age results in decreased healing;
2   genetics/skin type – darker-skinned people have a propensity to scar more, as do people with a family history of poor scarring/healing;
3   poor wound care – poor care of the wound after a biopsy or excision increases risk of infection, bleeding and poor edge alignment. These can prolong healing and lead to scarring. Good wound care and reducing the risk of scarring are discussed below;
4   infection – infection of the wound leads to further inflammation and destruction of viable, healthy tissue. This increases healing time and the risk of scarring;
5   anatomical location – areas such as the shoulders, feet, back and chest are under high tensile pressures. Wounds in these areas tend to heal slower and have an increased risk of producing thicker scars. Wounds located on the lower limbs also tend to heal more slowly;
6   lifestyle choices (e.g.smoking, alcohol, poor diet) – poor nutrition, a history of smoking and excess alcohol consumption can lead to delayed healing;
7   chronic disease (e.g. peripheral oedema, peripheral vascular disease, diabetes) – people with chronic diseases have an increased risk of infection and delayed wound healing due to the nature of their chronic illness. For example, diabetes reduces the body's natural ability to fight infections. Other illnesses that slow the natural healing process are those which lead to reduced blood flow to the healing tissues (e.g. peripheral oedema, which is chronic swelling of the legs, heart disease, liver disease or poor lymphatic drainage). It is also seen in peripheral vascular disease (reduced blood flow to the legs) as seen in people with heart disease and

smokers. Prevention and/or achieving optimal control of these conditions will improve scarring of any healing wound;

8   certain medications – some medications can interact with the body's natural wound repair mechanisms. It is important to discuss with your doctor any medications you are taking and whether any of them will affect your body's healing process.

Reducing the risks of scarring

There are a few risk factors for scarring that we cannot control, such as genetics, age and anatomical location. Certain other factors, however, can be addressed and minimised to reduce the appearance or formation of chronic scarring. These include proper post-biopsy wound care and lifestyle factors.

Post-biopsy skin care and management

To keep wet or dry?
Open wounds heal better in a moist environment.

Shave biopsies are best kept moist, with regular application of a film of Vaseline or another occlusive ointment. Occlusive ointment is ointment that stays on the surface of the skin and is not absorbed. Alternatively, some wound dressings are intended to keep the site moist. This helps prevent scab formation and provides a topical barrier to aid your skin's protection against infection.

Shave biopsies take approximately as long to heal as does a scraped knee, around one to two weeks.

Wounds closed with sutures are best kept dry; however, should a scab form, gently wash it away with warm salty water.

Preventing infection
After the first few days, daily cleaning of the wound site with warm soapy water will help prevent infection. The area should be patted dry, with minimal rubbing/trauma.

In the case of wounds closed with a suture, a topical adhesive dressing is often applied to protect and support the wound in its early healing stages.

Routine use of antibiotics to prevent infection is not currently recommended in low-risk, minor excisions. The overall incidence of infection following minor surgery in general practice in Australia is 2–9%.

Your doctor may choose to prescribe a topical or oral antibiotic if they consider you to be at high risk of infection.

Always wash your hands before touching any wounds!

Minimising tension along scar line

To help reduce the occurrence of increased tension along scar lines, it is important to avoid exercising or heavy lifting for at least 24–48 hours post biopsy or surgery. Your doctor may recommend a longer time of reduced activity, depending on the size and depth of your wound.

Topical lotions and concoctions

Application of topical vitamin E creams, antibacterial lotions or other gels/ointments to new wounds are generally not recommended given that they may in fact interfere with the healing process. Only in certain circumstances will your doctor recommend the application of an anti-inflammatory lotion to prevent infection. Otherwise, keeping your wound dry and/or using an occlusive dressing, including applications such as Vaseline, in the case of an open wound is appropriate.

Avoiding certain medications

Medications which prolong bleeding (e.g. aspirin, warfarin, clexane, NSAIDs) or others which may interfere with natural healing processes (e.g. corticosteroids) can in some cases prolong healing time. It is important to discuss your medications with your doctor. Please note: you should not stop taking these medications without your doctor's advice.

Addressing lifestyle

Eating a well balanced diet, maintaining a healthy weight range and avoiding cigarettes and excess alcohol will ensure your skin receives the appropriate nutrients it needs to heal itself to the best of its ability.

Appropriate monitoring and timely management of complications

It is important to have a basic understanding of how your wound should look during the healing process. Addressing any immediate complications or poor progress early is important in preventing longer-term complications and poor scar results. Danger signs and symptoms of poor wound healing include pain, bleeding, discharge, redness, pus, tenderness and older skin.

Continued reduction of tension along suture lines

Your doctor may recommend keeping your healing wound under constant low tension to prevent excessive forces along the suture line. This can be achieved with the application of an adhesive dressing perpendicular to the suture line, for two to four weeks.

Decrease sun exposure

New skin is especially sensitive to the sun and protective sun measures should be taken with any newly formed skin or scars (e.g. sun avoidance, daily sunscreen, zinc, clothing, hat).

Timely removal of sutures

Removing sutures too early or too late can affect the appearance of a scar. In general, sutures are removed after:

- face, 7 days;
- trunk, 10–14 days;
- legs, 14+ days.

It is important to remember that people with chronic health issues or a history of poor healing may need a longer period before sutures are removed.

Scar massage

It has been suggested that gentle massaging of a scar after sutures have been removed may help improve its aesthetic appearance. However, there is limited research in this area and most evidence is anecdotal.

Types of scarring

Unfortunately scar contractures, hypertrophic scarring and keloid scarring can arise, even in the case of a simple skin biopsy. All are described in detail below. Based on their location, these types of scars can lead to significant disfigurement, functional abnormalities and anxieties relating to their cosmetic appearance (Figs 11.33–11.35).

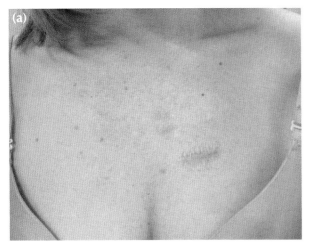
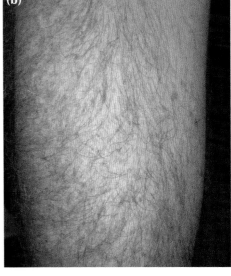

Fig. 11.33: (a) Healed scar on the chest. (b) Healed scar on the forearm.

Keloid and hypertrophic scarring is a result of abnormal responses to injury. In these situations, too much collagen has been deposited into the healing wound during the three basic stages of inflammatory wound repair.

The treatment of excess scarring is often managed by specialist dermatologists or surgeons. Treatment options include surgical and non-surgical means.

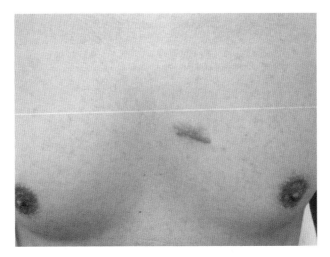

Fig. 11.34: A hypertrophic scar on the chest.

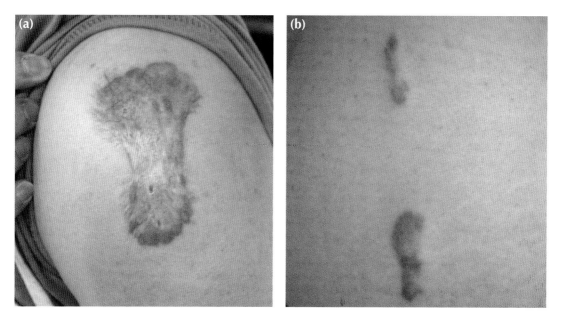

Fig. 11.35: Keloid scars.

Both types of scarring respond to the same treatment therapies. There is no one best-treatment option, and the large number of treatment options reflects that, often, these types of scars have a poor response or outcome.

Treatment options

Corticosteroid injections

This is the first-line therapy and involves injecting a solution of corticosteroid medication into the scar. The corticosteroid solution supresses (dampens down) the inflammatory process and increases vasoconstriction (compression of the small, new blood vessels) within the scar. It minimises the natural inflammatory process which forms scars, thus attempting to minimise the amount of collagen deposited in the wound. Usually, two to three injections are required over several months. Newer scars have a better prognosis than does the treatment of older, more established scars.

Silicone sheeting

This involves the topical application of a silicone sheet over the new scar. Newer options include silicone gels, foams, sprays and strips. It is thought that the silicone in these products increases the temperature and hydration of the developing scar, causing it to soften and flatten. For optimal results, it has been recommended that these sheets be applied 12–24 hours a day for up to two to three months.

Surgical removal

Unfortunately, surgical removal often only results in immediate satisfaction – given time, keloid scars usually recur. Surgical removal is thus often used in combination with other scar-reducing techniques.

Combination therapy

A combined method of surgical removal, with early introduction of corticosteroid injections or silicone sheeting, has been proposed as a method which produces better (reduced) scar recurrence rates.

Pulsed dye laser

This treatment modality is available only through specialised centres. It involves treating keloid scars with short-pulsed dye laser. Trials have reported reduced redness and improved skin texture. It can be quite costly and there is only limited evidence to support the technique.

Over-the-counter treatments

It is thought that the anti-oxidative properties of vitamin E would be beneficial in preventing scars. The evidence to support this is limited and the use of topical vitamin E cream can, in some circumstances, prevent healing. Some people may develop an acute contact dermatitis (irritation of the skin) which could delay healing, and it is thought that application of vitamin E too early can reduce the tensile strength of a scar. The use of creams during early stages of wound repair is therefore generally discouraged.

Are there differences between men and women?

Overall, men have both a higher incidence of and higher mortality rate from NMSCs. The lifetime risk of developing an NMSC is two in three men versus three in five women.

In Australia, 68% of the total 2000+ deaths from skin cancers (both NMSCs and melanomas) each year in Australia are men. Of the estimated 521 NMSC-related deaths in 2012, 362 were men and 159 were women.

Key points

- Keep your wound free from infection by cleaning it daily with a salt water solution.
- An open wound should be kept moist and a closed wound should be kept dry.
- Preventing the formation of thick dry scabs will help minimise scarring.
- Reduce tension along the suture line: minimise exercise and heavy lifting post biopsy or surgery.
- Monitor your healing wound and seek medical attention early if any complications arise.
- Maintain a healthy lifestyle: avoiding cigarettes and excess alcohol will improve healing outcomes.
- Ask your doctor if there are any medications (including over-the-counter) that you should use or avoid during the healing period.
- Thickened scars are more common in younger, darker-skinned people and in areas under high tension (shoulder, chest, upper back).
- Although available, treatment options for thickened scars are limited in effectiveness. An informed choice is essential when considering them.

The locations of BCCs and SCCs on the body also vary between the sexes. Given that around 99% of NMSCs are caused by accumulated sun exposure, the variation of location between the sexes mirrors the differences in the body areas chronically exposed to the sun.

The anatomical distribution for BCCs are similar for men and women (Fig. 11.36). The anatomical distribution for SCCs varies between men and women (Fig. 11.37).

What to ask your doctor when diagnosed with a skin cancer

- What type of skin cancer do I have?
- What are my treatment options?
- What should I expect from treatment?
- What are the side effects of the treatment?
- What scarring should I expect and what can I do to minimise scarring?

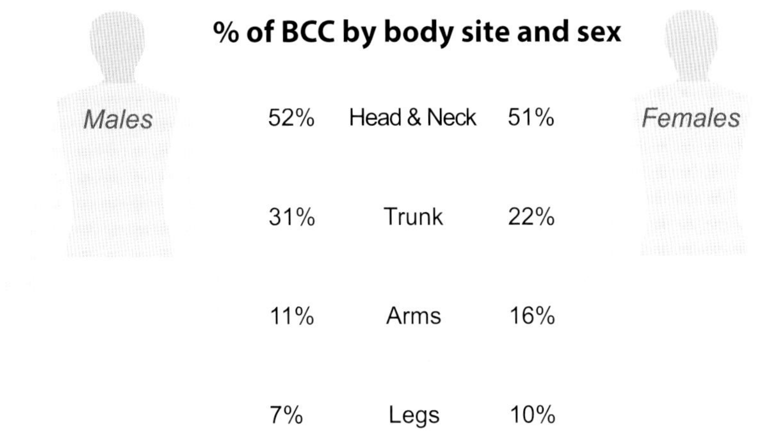

% of BCC by body site and sex

	Males			Females
	52%	Head & Neck	51%	
	31%	Trunk	22%	
	11%	Arms	16%	
	7%	Legs	10%	

Fig. 11.36: Anatomical distribution of BCCs, men and women. With permission of Cancer Council Victoria.

- What are the 'danger signs' I should look out for during the recovery period after treatment?
- How should I care for my skin – daily?
- How should I care for my skin following a biopsy or excision?

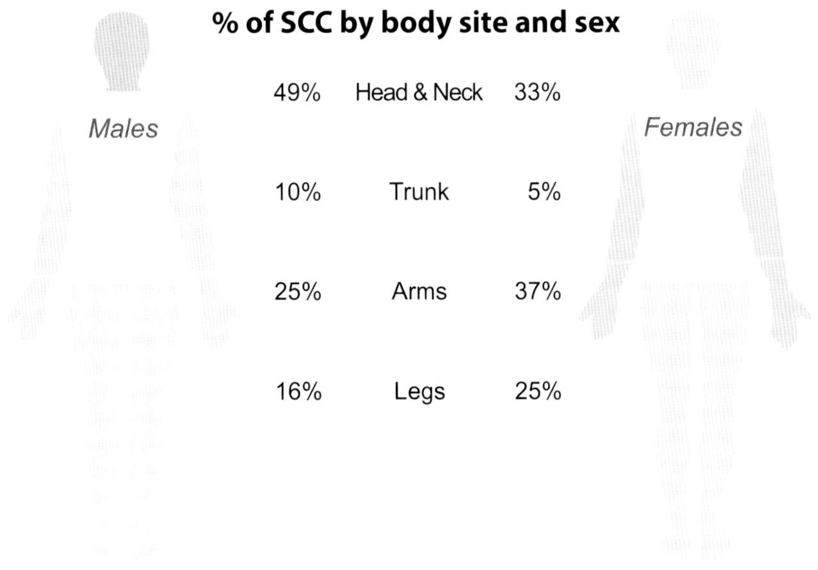

% of SCC by body site and sex

	Males			Females
	49%	Head & Neck	33%	
	10%	Trunk	5%	
	25%	Arms	37%	
	16%	Legs	25%	

Fig. 11.37: Anatomical distribution of SCCs, men and women. With permission of Cancer Council Victoria.

- Vitamin D: how much sun exposure do I need?
- What are the recovery rates, i.e. how effective is my treatment likely to be?
- What are the chances of the cancer recurring?
- When do I need to see you again?

You must also inform your doctor if you have a tendency to scar.

Further reading

Cancer Council Australia (2008) Basal cell carcinoma, squamous cell carcinoma (and related lesions): a guide to clinical management in Australia. Canstat no.44, Skin Cancer. Cancer Council, Victoria.

Cancer Council Victoria (2013) Sunsmart statistics and statements.

Heal C, Buettner P, Browning S (2006) Risk factors for wound infection after minor surgery in general practice. *Medical Journal of Australia* **185**(5), 255–258.

Juckett G (2009) Hartman-Adams: management of keloids and hypertrophic scars. *American Family Physician* **80**(3), 253–260.

Lathlean S (1999) Skin cancer in general practice in South Australia: a five-year study. *Australian Family Physician* **28** (Suppl. 1), S28–S31.

Shin TM, Bordeaux JS (2012) The role of massage in scar management: a literature review. *Dermatologic Surgery* **38**(3), 414–423.

Chapter 12

What about after skin cancer treatment?

Jamie von Nida and Jonathan Chan

Key messages

- After skin cancer has been treated successfully, you need to be alert to the fact that you are at greater risk of additional cancers developing.
- You should know exactly what type of skin cancer you had and how it was treated. This will be important in talking to doctors in the future.
- Regular self-examinations looking for signs of skin cancer should become routine – at least every two months. Regular follow-up visits to your doctor are also important.
- Talk to your family about your skin cancer experience and encourage them to follow your example by being extra careful about sun protection.

Introduction

Once a skin cancer has been diagnosed and treated, optimal after-care depends on several factors. These include the type of cancer and the type of management, and an understanding of the prognosis and required ongoing care.

In this chapter, we will discuss and answer some common questions.

Is there an increased risk for other cancers?

Patients who have developed a skin cancer are at higher risk of developing further skin malignancies. Almost half the people diagnosed with basal cell carcinoma will develop a second BCC within three years. The three-year cumulative risk of developing another SCC or BCC is 10 times that of the comparable general population. A large study of 46 237 white men (who were followed from 1986 to 2008) and 107 339 women (1984–2008) indicated that apart from this increased risk of developing another NMSC, patients were also more likely to get other types of cancers. Males were slightly more likely to develop prostate cancer (relative risk 1.11, i.e. 11% more likely than a man who has not had an NMSC) and about double the chance of getting melanoma. Females with an NMSC were at 19% higher risk of developing breast cancer, 32% increased chance of lung cancer, 30% higher risk of leukaemia, one and a half times higher chance of kidney cancer and two and a half times greater risk of melanoma.

Although the higher rate of melanoma can be linked to sun exposure, it is difficult to explain why the rate of other malignancies is increased in patients with skin cancer. The authors of the large study suggested that patients might be genetically predisposed to cancers and hence have a higher rate of all malignancies, not just cutaneous ones.

Patients with melanoma are over 10 times more likely to get another melanoma. Greater risk of developing another melanoma was seen in males and among people diagnosed with a first melanoma under the age of 30. Similarly to non-melanoma skin cancers, patients with primary melanoma were more likely to develop breast or prostate cancer.

How often do I need to go back to the doctor?

It is recommended that all patients who have had a skin cancer removed should have an annual skin review to look for new lesions. Some patients who are developing multiple skin cancers or frequent skin cancers or who are immunosuppressed may require more frequent reviews, perhaps every three or six months. The aim of these reviews is to detect lesions at an early stage where they may be easier to treat and surgery may be avoided.

Patients who have had a malignant melanoma cut out will require regular follow-up by the doctor. The frequency of reviews is dependent on the stage of the tumour. People who had thicker lesions will require three-monthly reviews for a year, then six-monthly reviews for two years and then yearly reviews. At the reviews the doctor will examine the entire skin surface and review the sites of previous surgery. They may also examine lymph nodes or other areas.

There is always a risk that the skin cancer may recur at the site of excision, where the original cancer was. There are many factors which influence the risk of recurrence. They include the type of treatment used, what previous treatments were applied, location on the body, size of the tumour, depth of tumour invasion, tumour type and whether there was evidence of nerve invasion, what the cause of the cancer might have been (especially if it was not UV exposure) and the extent to which the immune system has been damaged or suppressed.

The risk of recurrence for a surgically removed BCC is low, 4–9%. The risk of recurrence for an SCC which has been cut out is 5–19%. The risk of recurrence for surgically excised melanoma has recently been shown to be 8%.

What should I look for?

Patients who have had previous skin malignancies should undertake self-examination on a regular basis. Every two months is wise, to try and detect any new lesions early. Tips on what to look for are covered in Chapter 9. Patients should pay particular attention to lesions that are getting bigger, bleeding (with minor trauma or spontaneously), developing multiple colours or becoming symptomatic (itching, tender, painful).

As a general rule, a lesion that does not heal within three weeks is a skin malignancy unless proven otherwise.

What should I need to know from my doctor?

The type of skin cancer is often confusing for the patient. The diagnosis of the type of cancer can have important implications, particularly with ongoing follow-up and for patients transferring care to another doctor. For example, a completely excised nodular BCC on the forehead will have the same scar as a 1.4 mm thick invasive melanoma that was excised in the area. The prognosis of the melanoma, however, is significantly worse and has implications for ongoing follow-up and assessment of further risk of skin cancer. So it is important that, after the diagnosis of the skin cancer, you obtain the histology report as well as an understanding of the prognosis and long-term implications of the cancer. It is also a good idea to remember the type of skin cancer you had removed, as this might become important later.

What other problems should I worry about?

Depression

Studies have demonstrated that significant psychological stresses occur with the diagnosis of skin cancer. An overwhelming theme was concern at ongoing sun exposure and the need for sun avoidance. Another significant concern was the likelihood for the cancer to spread or recur. In addition, 7% of patients in a German study had anxiety scores that indicated they needed professional help and 17% had post-traumatic symptoms, i.e. those patients had enough anxiety to indicate a diagnosis of post-traumatic stress disorder. It has been estimated that one third of patients with melanoma report increased mental distress.

This indicates that although most patients deal with their skin cancer well, a significant proportion experience anxiety and depression.

It is therefore not unusual for a patient to feel anxious or depressed with the treatment or the diagnosis of skin cancer. Talk about your feelings with your doctor. In addition, there are many organisations that provide cancer support networks.

Life insurance

The policies of many life insurance companies in Australia have melanoma clauses. Some companies will pay a lump sum on the diagnosis of any invasive melanoma despite the depth or severity of the disease. Other companies will pay out and limit benefits once the diagnosis of melanoma has been made. The ability to obtain a policy may be limited or the premiums increased after a diagnosis of melanoma regardless of the severity of the disease.

Can I give blood?

The Australian Red Cross Service excludes any person who had a cancer, including invasive melanoma, from donating blood for five years after diagnosis and treatment of the skin cancer.

What should I tell my family?

The greatest risk of melanoma occurs in patients who have a first-degree relative with melanoma and who have multiple irregular moles. So it is essential to inform first-degree relatives (mother, father, brother, sister, son or daughter) after a diagnosis of melanoma. Relatives should discuss the family history of melanoma with their local doctor.

What about vitamin D levels?

Some types of skin cancers are due to cumulative solar exposure over a lifetime, so it is logical that patients who have had a skin cancer should try to minimise further solar damage to their skin. They should stay out of the sun or adopt sun protection strategies such as wearing sun protective clothing and broad-brimmed hats as well as sunscreen (SPF30 or higher). The detailed sun protection advice earlier in this book is of great importance to skin cancer patients and their family after a lesion has been treated. Many people are concerned, however, that they will become vitamin D deficient if they avoid the sun completely. In most areas of Australia people can achieve adequate vitamin D levels with only 10 minutes exposure to the face and back of the hands at 9a.m. in summer. More detail on vitamin D is found in Chapter 8.

Conclusion

Once you have had a skin cancer diagnosis, things change a little. The signal is that you are unfortunately a little more vulnerable to a future cancer diagnosis. If you are the first in your family to have skin cancer, it also sends a signal to those who are closest to you, that they too might be at higher risk of skin cancer.

Learning more about the technical aspects of sun protection, establishing wise sun protection habits and establishing a regular regime of skin-checking and check-ups with your doctor at appropriate intervals will help reduce the chance of additional and more serious disease down the track.

Chapter 13

What we are doing about sun protection: are we making progress?

Suzanne Dobbinson and Terry Slevin

Key messages

- Substantial shifts in people's attitudes and use of sun protection have occurred in recent decades in Australia.
- Tanning is less popular and desirable than it was eight years ago and both adults and adolescents are reporting being sunburned less frequently than a decade ago.
- The fashions at times promote brief clothing, tanned skin and intentional sun exposure.
- Skin cancer prevention programs and mass media campaigns have a role in balancing these less supportive messages in the social environment. Greater commitment to skin cancer prevention remains essential.
- There is still room and need for improvements in the use of covering clothing and hats. Our increased use of hats and reduction in sun exposure might quickly be eroded if we don't continue to act on and be aware of the need for skin cancer prevention.
- A better understanding of the technical aspects of UV radiation will help in making good sun protection choices.

Introduction

In Australia there has been public action on skin cancer for over 30 years, resulting in significant shifts in our awareness of skin cancer and the need for sun protection. Action included a range of campaigns, programs and research to reduce people's exposure to UV radiation (UVR) through public education, mass media, policy and legislative changes to support sun protection. Advertising skin cancer prevention messages during summer has been particularly important in setting the agenda and prompting increased sun protection. Similar programs have run in New Zealand since 1988.

Slip! Slop! Slap! was the first advertisement to be broadcast across Australia with the now-iconic cartoon character Sid Seagull, who sang messages about sun protection. Many other skin cancer prevention advertisements followed, including a national campaign run by the Australian government from 2006 to 2010. The messages have become more graphic and often include images that depict the severe consequences of skin cancer, as well as messages and images that target our attitudes to tanning.

These campaign messages helped counteract other images and messages in the broader social environment that were less supportive of people's use of covering clothing and hats. In the early 1980s, tans were typically darker. From the 1960s and 1970s it was not only more acceptable but also more fashionable for more skin to be on show, so briefer and less sun protective clothes became normal.

Although our awareness of skin cancer and the need to protect from UVR increased over the decades, fashion trends did not always follow the changing attitudes. At times, fashions for darker tans made a resurgence. A review of images in women's magazines from 1987 to 2005 found relatively few models were portrayed wearing hats (11% of images). Photographs of models in beach settings commonly had dark tans and lots of visible skin – these images promoted increased sun exposure. In contrast, the clothes worn by most actors in youth-oriented Australian film covered their arms and legs; a few wore hats.

Influential role models were targeted by prevention programs. Sponsorship and policy change by the surf lifesaving movement transformed the 'bronzed Aussie lifesaver' in some Australian states into a role model for good sun protection. Lifesavers now wear long sleeves and broad-brimmed hats when on patrol. Sports celebrities were also recruited to promote the sun protection message in high-profile outdoor summer sports (Fig. 13.1).

Advocacy and support for policies promoting sun protection at schools have had far-reaching benefits. The SunSmart schools program helped schools shift their uniform policies from

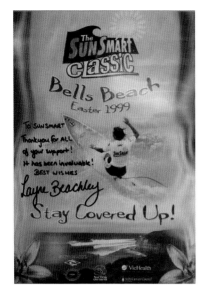
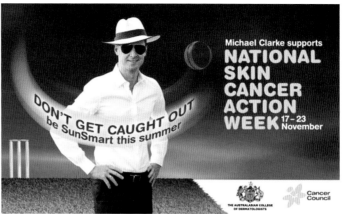

Fig. 13.1: High-profile sports celebrities can help promote the sun protection message.

baseball caps to broad-brimmed hats and from short-sleeved to longer-sleeved shirts. Sun protection policies are in place in most schools and early childhood centres. These policies have also driven an increase in the amount of shade available in school playgrounds, including more covered outdoor learning areas (COLAs, see Chapter 6).

While primary school children are generally more compliant with sun protection policies and practices promoted by parents and teachers, concerns about adolescents remain. But there is good evidence that shade in high school grounds will be well accepted and used by teenagers without any need for enforcement policies. The next challenge is to ensure that shade is incorporated in high school upgrades and plans for new high schools.

Other trends in the uptake of sun protection include increased use of swimwear covering the back and shoulders (e.g. 'rashies') especially among children, and provision of shade over toddlers' wading pools.

Australian workplaces are also taking action to prevent ~200 melanomas and 34 000 non-melanoma skin cancers per year attributed to occupational UVR exposures. Since 2003, sun protection products have been a tax-deductible work expense for employees.

There has been some increase in the number of workplaces with sun protection policies: 57% of employed adults reported their workplaces had a sun protection policy in 2010–11 compared with 51% in 2003–04. However, in 2010–11 most employed adults still had to provide their own hat. About 45% of employed adults working at least some time outdoors reported their workplace provided hats. Safe Work Australia is currently revising its guidance notes to strengthen UV protection recommendations for workplaces.

This change in sun protection practices in workplaces has also been driven by an increase in compensation payments for skin cancer linked to occupational exposure. In the last 10 years in Australia, about $4 million per year has been paid out to workers who, due at least in part to unprotected sun exposure at work, have had skin cancers diagnosed and treated. About 150 cases per year are successfully claiming compensation.

Have people in Australia changed how much skin they protect?

The pattern of improvement in sun protection behaviours (hats and sunscreen) in Victoria, where surveys have run longest, shows two distinct periods. First, during the early 1990s with rapid improvements in sun protection. The second period had more variable changes in sun protection. There was a similar pattern of improvement in the reported proportion of the body with unprotected skin (not covered by clothing, hats and sunscreen) when outdoors on summer weekends. The pattern of change was similar across age groups.

The national surveys record changes in Australians' use of sun protection for the past decade. Although there were reductions in weekend sunburn during this period, there was little positive change in hat-wearing among both adolescents and adults. However, there were some increases in adults wearing long-sleeved tops and using sunscreen. Less time was spent outdoors, and this was consistent with the reduction in sunburn incidence. Among adolescents the reduction in reported weekend sunburn was consistent with fewer adolescents spending time outdoors during peak UVR hours.

This may have been driven by sun protection intention, or it might simply result from a move towards increased use of screen-based indoor entertainment or the particularly wet summer in 2010–11 on the east coast.

Who wears hats, protective clothes and sunscreen, and who doesn't?

The Cancer Council's national sun protection survey provides comparable assessment of Australians' use of hats and other sun protection behaviours. The prevalence of children's, adolescents' and adults' sun protection behaviours during peak UVR hours on summer weekends are described in Table 13.1. These data highlight that the majority of children were well protected compared with adolescents and adults. This is encouraging, as early exposure to UVR increases the lifetime skin cancer risk.

A hat was the most common form of sun protection used by children and adolescents when outdoors, but more adults wore sunglasses than hats.

Very few Australians in any age group wore tops with at least three-quarter length sleeves on summer weekends. Approximately one in three children and adults, but only one in five adolescents, stayed under shade during outdoor activity on the weekend. Increased use of shade would be beneficial, as shade use and spending less time outdoors are commonly associated with reduced risk of sunburn.

Overall, significantly more adults use hats and covering clothing than adolescents. Adolescents were less likely than adults to have worn any hat, a wide-brimmed hat, three-quarter sleeved tops, or stayed under shade. More adolescents than adults spent time outdoors during peak UVR hours.

The surveys suggest there is a steep decline in the use of protective clothing during adolescence and into young adulthood – a time when fashion sense and a heightened focus on appearance and social concerns guide our choices. Older adults, who have experience with sunburn and are aware of skin damage, generally return to increased use of hats and protective clothing (Fig. 13.2).

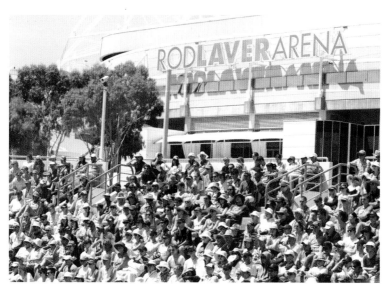

Fig. 13.2: Hats and clothing worn at the Australian Open tennis in Melbourne during January. Image courtesy of Tennis Australia.

Table 13.1: Prevalence of Australian's sun protection behaviours in summer (as measured by Cancer Council Australia's National Sun Protection surveys)

Reported behaviours on the weekend before the survey	Children* (0–11 years) 2003–04 N = 1140 (%)	Adolescents (12–17 years) 2003–04 N = 699 (%)	Adolescents (12–17 years) 2010–11 N = 1367 (%)	Adults (18–69 years) 2003–04 N = 5073 (%)	Adults (18–69 years) 2010–11 N = 5412 (%)
Outdoors (for more than 15 min)	73	80	77	73	66
Time (mins) during main outdoor activity in peak UVR	110	109.7	112	118.9	111
Sun protection used (during outdoor activity Sunday/Saturday)	N = 794	N = 561	N = 1047	N = 3683	N = 3583
Hat (headwear including caps, hats with narrow and wide brims)	64	38	23	48	45
Sunglasses	11	23	24	55	57
Stayed mostly under shade	32	19	21	27	28
Wore 3/4 or long-sleeved top	18	11	11	18	19
Wore 3/4 or long leg cover	29	37	28	46	44
Used SPF ≥15 sunscreen	58	37	37	33	36

Source: Volkov *et al.* (2013); Dobbinson *et al.* (2012).

* Survey data for children were from parent's reports of their children's behaviours. This survey component was included only in the 2003–04 survey.

National surveys show hats were more commonly worn by males than females at all ages. Among children, boys were more likely to wear a hat than girls but they were less likely to stay under shade during their outdoor activities. Boys also stayed outdoors in peak UVR for longer.

During adolescence, except for more hat use by boys than girls, there was little difference in sun protection by gender. Distinctive patterns emerged only among adults. On summer weekends more men wore a hat than women when outdoors between 11am and 3pm. More women than men wore covering clothing on their arms and legs, used sunscreen, wore sunglasses and stayed mostly under shade. Women also spent significantly less time outdoors during these peak UVR hours.

These differences contribute to a higher incidence of sunburn on summer weekends among boys and men than among girls and women. Adolescents' incidence of sunburn was similar and high for both sexes. These recent surveys may well reflect long-term preferences for sun protection among men and women, which may explain why the skin cancer rates in men are much greater than the skin cancer rate in women.

What are the barriers to sun protection?

What is considered 'normal' and fashionable is most likely to drive the choice of hats worn by males. In 2010–11, 51% of men compared with 36% of women wore some style of hat when outside on a typical summer weekend, but only 23% of men and 19% of women wore a wide-brimmed hat which would offer more sun protection. Research in the 1980s found men and women showed little difference in their intentions to wear hats. The main factors influencing hat use by both sexes were inconvenience and fear of spoiling their hairstyle.

Other factors were the beliefs that hats were uncomfortable and caused baldness, deterring use. Those who believed that wearing hats prevented eyestrain, sunburn and skin cancer were more encouraged to do so. Males were more likely to mention several other issues with hats, including problems playing sport, getting a sweaty head, the hat being a nuisance on windy days, the difficulty of finding one that fit properly, expense, and being self-conscious in a hat.

Anecdotally, concern about 'hat hair' may be more of a barrier to hat-wearing for women. However, the national surveys show women (45%) more commonly used sunscreen on summer weekends than men (29%). In Australia in recent years the majority of moisturisers sold for women include an SPF of 15+, often marketed as anti-ageing. Women may choose to use sunscreens or moisturiser with a sunscreen component as an alternative to wearing a hat but, depending on the extent of the moisturiser use, this may leave the ears and neck vulnerable to excessive UV exposure where hairstyles are short.

Recent research on adolescents' attitudes to hat-wearing and sun protection showed that hat-hair and problems with sport were a concern and deterred them from hat use. However, adolescents' comments suggested that hats, clothing and sunglasses were worn more to create a fashion image than for sun protection. Adolescents' desire for a tan was also a significant barrier to hat-wearing. Several of the early SunSmart ads focused on hats as fashionable and normal, to counter beliefs that hat-wearing made people self-conscious and to promote awareness of the benefits of reduced sunburn and skin cancer prevention. These campaigns were shown to be effective in increasing the likelihood of people wearing a hat on summer weekends. In summer weeks when there was more campaign advertising (as indicated by TARPs, a standard measure of TV audience exposure to ads) there was an increase in the number of people using sun protection. For example, more people wore a hat outdoors than after weekends with less campaign advertising.

TV advertising may be helpful in providing timely reminders for sun protection during summer months, as well as making use of hats and covering clothing more acceptable. For adolescents, rules about sun protection made by parents, teachers and coaches also encourage hat use. Sun protection and skin cancer prevention messages reach all age groups through community-wide initiatives via many channels and settings.

The influence of temperature and weather on sun protection practice

Understandably, the most dominant influence on our choice of clothing is the weather. When it is hot we want to wear less clothing so as to stay cool, when the temperature is cold we cover up to stay warm. Rain and wind also prompt more protective clothing, again to stay warm and dry.

For that reason it is important to factor in the temperature and weather of the days for which sun protection information was reported. This is a routine feature of large surveys and it allows a more meaningful understanding of the sun protection behaviour changes reported over time.

Encouragingly, these surveys show that although people wore less clothing on summer weekends when the weather was hot, adults were also prompted to use sun protection (wear hats, sunscreen and stay in the shade). However, this protection was not enough to offset a higher percentage of adults and adolescents being sunburned on weekend days above 22°C. Additional weather effects were that clear skies prompted use of sunglasses by adults, and sunburn rates increased slightly overall on days with less cloud cover.

Since efforts to promote skin cancer prevention have been more prominent, there is a greater trend for people to be reminded to protect their skin when the weather is very hot. The feeling of heat on the skin is a physical reminder of the 'burning effect of the sun'. This feeling of heat likely promotes the increase in use of hats, sunscreen and shade.

However, despite all the influences of other weather factors on people's behaviours, we should remember that exposure to UVR is the cause of sunburn and skin cancer. Chapter 2 described how the UV Index, the measure of the intensity of the UV radiation, is not always aligned with the temperature over summer months. The UV Index can easily reach the extreme range of 11 or 12 anywhere in Australia during summer, no matter whether the temperature is 27°C or 37°C. A cooler day can easily follow a very hot day, while the UV Index might be almost exactly the same for the two consecutive days. People can suffer severe burning on cooler days if they do not protect their skin.

What are we doing when we get sunburned?

In the summer of 2003–04 18% of adults and 25% of adolescents reported being sunburned in the most recent weekend. Those figures fell to 13% of adults and 21% of adolescents in 2010–11. So the figures are heading in the right direction but more effort is needed, particularly by adolescents.

The most common reasons people gave for being burned were that they forgot their sun protection (hats, sunscreen), the sunscreen was not applied and reapplied thoroughly, or they were out in the sun too long.

Due to higher reflection of UVR and the typically brief clothing we wear around water, being at the beach or the pool or doing water sports without taking care to protect from the sun is a recipe for sunburn. However, even though water-related activities are risky for sunburn, because more people are outdoors doing non-aquatic activities like everyday routines, gardening and housework, or in the backyard, most sunburn is from incidental exposure to the sun.

Knowing this gives us clues as to where we need to 'lift our game'.

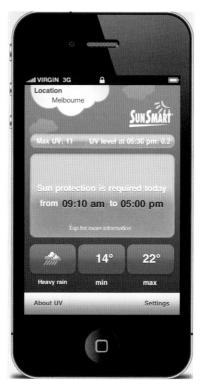

Fig. 13.3: The SunSmart app gives live local UV Index information to aid sun protection.

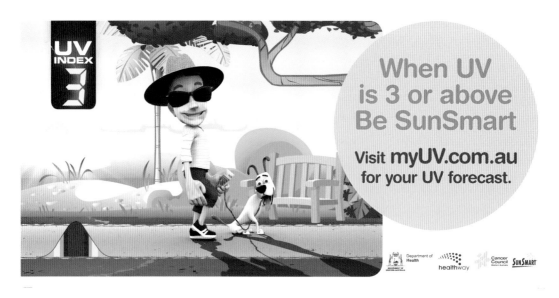

Fig. 13.4: An image from the Cancer Council WA UV Index campaign in the summer of 2012–13.

What more can be done to promote good sun protection behaviours?

Clearly there are many options that are effective in achieving good sun protection – better use of hats and clothing, creating and using more shade, using sunscreen. But they are only useful if we remember to use them – at the right time and in the right place. Timely advertising messages through summer can be reminders but other strategies are also important, as is other support for sun protection e.g. policies encouraging use of sun protection in schools and workplaces, provision of shade at outdoor venues. Web-based information from popular news sites and weather information channels, as well as SMS, smartphone apps (Fig. 13.3) and well located signs at beaches and outdoor recreation locations are all being employed to encourage sun protection when the UV Index is 3 and above.

We need to improve people's understanding of UVR and how geographical location, the time of day and the time of year influence the UV level. The UV Index (Chapter 2) is a measure of UV and can be used as a guide to prompt when sun protection is needed.

A recent campaign in Western Australia aims to improve community understanding and use of the UV Index (Fig. 13.4). While it is too early to measure its impact on skin cancer rates, early signs are encouraging. Prior to the campaign 7% of people knew that a UV Index level of 3 signalled the need for sun protection. After one summer of the campaign the figure had risen to 29% (among those who were aware of the campaign). The campaign will run for three summers.

No doubt many more good ideas for skin cancer programs will continue to prompt us to cover up at the right place and the right time, and reduce our skin cancer risk. Greater investment in such campaigns is important if the efforts are to influence the choices of Australians and New Zealanders.

Further reading

Dobbinson S, Wakefield M, Hill D, Girgis A, Aitken JF, Beckmann K, Reeder AI, Herd N, Spittal MJ, Fairthorne A, Bowles KA (2012) Children's sun-exposure and sun protection: prevalence in Australia and related parental factors. *Journal of the American Academy of Dermatology* **66**(6), 938–947.

Volkov A, Dobbinson S, Wakefield M, Slevin T (2013) Seven-year trends in sun protection and sunburn among Australian adolescents and adults. *Australia and New Zealand Journal of Public Health* **37**(1), 63–69.

Glossary

ABCDE checklist   This is a mnemonic device that uses the initials of key aspects of spots on the skin that may indicate the presence of skin cancer. Does skin spot or lesion look like it is **A**symmetrical, does it have an irregular **B**order, does it contain different **C**olours, is it changing **D**iameter or is it **E**volving or changing in size, shape or colour ?

Basal cell   A small round cell found in the lower part (or base) of the epidermis, the outer layer of the skin.

Basal cell carcinoma (BCC)   Cancer or carcinoma in the basal cell of the skin. BCCs generally remain within the basal cells. The most common but generally least dangerous form of skin cancer.

Benign   A non-cancerous lesion.

BRAF   This gene makes a protein called B-Raf which is involved in sending signals inside cells causing cell growth. This gene signals melanoma cells to multiply and is present in about half of all melanoma cases.

Breslow thickness   A measure of how many millimetres in depth the melanoma has spread into the skin.

Carotenoids   A yellow, red or orange substance found mostly in plants, including carrots, sweet potatoes and dark green leafy vegetables, and in many fruits, grains and oils. Some carotenoids are changed into vitamin A in the body and some are being studied in the prevention of cancer. A carotenoid is a type of antioxidant.

Dermis   The inner layer of the two main layers of the skin (between the epidermis and subcutaneous tissue).

DNA   The molecules inside cells that carry genetic information and pass it from one generation to the next. DNA is the acronym for **D**eoxyribo**N**ucleic **A**cid.

Epidermis   The outer layer of the two main layers of the skin. The layer beneath the epidermis is the dermis.

Epidermodysplasia verruciformis (EV)   A rare hereditary skin disorder associated with a high risk of skin cancer, characterised by an abnormal susceptibility to human papillomavirus (HPV).

Erythema   The clinical terms for a sunburn or reddening of the skin due to UV exposure.

Excise/excision   Cutting out a skin lesion. This allows the lesion to be examined under the microscope to make a final diagnosis.

Fitzpatrick classification   A classification scheme for skin, based upon the skin's burning and tanning responses. The fairest types of skin are level 1 and the darkest types of skin are level 6.

Freckles   Brownish spots on the skin that are due to melanin production and that increase in number and intensity following exposure to sunlight.

Gene   The basic unit of heredity. A gene is a sequence of nucleotides in a segment of DNA that provides the 'blueprint' for all proteins in the body.

Histopathologist   A specialist doctor who examines human tissue and diagnoses the presence or absence of cancer or other diseases.

Human papillomavirus (HPV)   A very large group of viruses that infect human cells. Many are apparently harmless, but some cause warts (e.g. common warts, plantar warts, genital warts) and others cause cancers of the cervix, vulva, vagina, anus and throat. Certain strains of HPV have been implicated in squamous cell carcinomas of the skin.

Incidence   A measure of frequency of diseases. Strictly, an incidence is a rate, and is expressed in terms of the numbers of people newly affected by a disease, per unit of population, per year.

In situ   In its original position or place. For example, the term 'carcinoma in situ' refers to cancerous cells found only in the place where they first formed. They have not spread to deeper layers.

Keratinocyte   An epidermal cell that produces keratin (a fibrous protein). These are the most commonly found cells in the epidermis.

Lesion   An area of skin which does not resemble the surrounding areas. It may be a growth or simply a patch of skin.

Local anaesthetic   An injection to numb the skin.

Lymph nodes   These form part of the body's lymphatic system and act as filters, trapping cancer cells including melanoma.

Lymphoma   A type of cancer that arises from cells of the immune system.

Margin of excision   An amount of healthy skin around the edge of the excision. The purpose of a margin is to ensure all cancer cells are removed, while aiming to minimise the amount of healthy skin removed.

Melanin   A pigment that is produced in a group of cells known as melanocytes. It gives colour to the skin and eyes and helps protect the skin from damage by ultraviolet light.

Melanocyte   A cell in the skin and eyes that produces the pigment called melanin.

Melanoma   Sometimes referred to as Cutaneous Malignant Melanoma (CMM), this is the potentially most dangerous form of skin cancer and can grow and spread rapidly. The cancer starts in the melanocytes.

Merkel cells   A cell type found directly below the epidermis. These cells are very close to the nerve endings that receive the sensation of touch and may be involved in touch.

Mitosis   The process by which a single parent cell divides to make two new daughter cells. Each daughter cell receives a complete set of chromosomes from the parent cell. This process allows the body to grow and replace cells.

Mutation   A permanent change in the DNA code of a gene. Genetic mutations can change the behaviour of a cell, making it prone to cancer.

Mole   A benign (non-cancer) growth (naevus) on the skin that is formed by a cluster of melanocytes. A naevus is usually dark and may be protrude above the skin surface.

Naevus   The medical term for a mole. The plural of naevus is naevi.

Non Melanoma Skin Cancer (NMSC)   Also sometimes referred to as Keratinocyte Cancers (KCs) is the collective name for skin cancers that are not melanoma. They are generally less likely to cause death but are far more common than melanoma and the large majority are either BCCs or SCCs.

Psoriasis   A chronic skin disease marked by red patches covered by white scales.

Radiation   Energy radiated in the form of waves or particles.

Selenium   A mineral that the body needs to stay healthy. It is found especially in grains and meat and is a type of antioxidant.

Solarium   A non-medical device that emits ultraviolet light for the purpose of creating a cosmetic tanning of the skin.

Squamous cell   A cell of or derived from the squamous epithelium (resembles scales or plates). These cells form the surface of the skin.

Squamous cell carcinoma (SCC)   Skin cancer that forms in the squamous cells of the skin. These are less common than BCCs and can spread to other parts of the body, and in extreme cases can cause death.

Standard Erythemal Dose (SED)   A measure of the UV dose of sunlight that results in sunburn; it requires an exposure of about 2 SED to produce a very mild sunburn in sun-sensitive individuals who burn easily and never tan. Technically an SED is 100 Joules/square metre.

Sun Protection Factor (SPF)   The measure of the level of protection provided by a sunscreen. The higher the SPF the higher the level of protection, measured by the multiple of the time spent in the sun before burning.

Surgical excision   Cutting out a skin lesion.

Sutured   Stitched; usually applying to stitching skin together after surgery or an injury.

Ultraviolet Protection Factor (UPF)   The measure of the level of protection provided by clothing. The higher the UPF the higher the level of protection, measured by the multiple of the time spent in the sun before burning.

Ultraviolet radiation   Electromagnetic radiation with wavelengths shorter than visible light, for which the primary source is the sun. Ultraviolet radiation that reaches the Earth's surface is made up of two types, UVA (longer wavelengths) and UVB (shorter wavelengths). Ultraviolet radiation also comes from artificial sources including sun lamps, tanning beds, medical sources and arc-welding.

Virus   The simplest infectious organism. Viruses are made up only of DNA or RNA, and have to live within the cells of another organism to reproduce. Some viruses damage the DNA of their host cells, causing mutations which can lead to cancer.

Xeroderma pigmentosum (XP)   A genetic condition characterised by the development of pigment abnormalities and multiple skin cancers in body areas exposed to the sun.

Index

medications, and increased sun
  sensitivity   56–7
Mediterranean building design   100
Mediterranean diet   133
melanin   2, 57, 151
melanocytes   2, 11, 22
melanoma apps   172
melanomas   xvi, 4
  advanced, treatment approaches   181–2
  age factors   11
  appearance   4, 166–7
  body sites   4, 12, 14, 22, 124, 162–3,
    166–7
  Breslow thickness of   174
  Clark level depth of invasion   174
  deaths from   6, 157
  diagnostic accuracy   170
  early detection   157
  early surgery   173–5
  family implications   182–3, 235
  from solaria   16, 48, 61
  in situ, thin and early stage   7
  incidence in fair-skinned populations living
    in different parts of the world   9–11
  of the inner eye   124
  and life insurance claims   234
  and lymph nodes   175, 176–7
  in men and women   xx, 8, 11–12
  and moles   22, 162–3, 166–7
  new technologies in diagnosis   171–2
  people who survive at least five years after
    diagnosis by 'stage'   158
  prevalence   5–6
  prevention through sunscreen use   92–3
  referral to a specialist   171
  and regular skin checks   170–1, 175
  stages of disease   158, 178–80

sunlight as major cause   13–14
surgical excision   173–5, 180
tests to determine spread   176–8
treatment   173–83
trends over time   6–8
what to ask your doctor   183
men
  barriers to hat use   243
  BCC and SCC incidence and location on
    the body   227–8, 229
  melanoma incidence   xx, 8, 11–12
  and risk of BCCs   187
  skin cancer rate   xix–xx
  sun protection   243
mental health, and vitamin D   147
Merkel cell carcinomas   4–5
Merkel cells   4
Mohs micrographic surgery   190, 208–9
molecular testing of melanoma
  specimens   178
moles   21–2
  ABCDE checklist   162
  appearance   164–7
  assessment with a dermatoscope   168
  benign   164
  and melanomas   22, 162–3, 166–7, 172
  seven-point checklist (7-PC)   162–3
  smartphone technology for self-
    assessment   172
  'ugly duckling' sign   163
Montreal Protocol   33
morphoeic BCCs   190
multiple sclerosis (MS)   145, 146
mutations   3–4, 13, 23, 24
  following UV radiation   15
  melanomas   178
myopia   125